D1036054

Handbook of Psychiatric Drugs

2008 Edition

Lawrence J. Albers, MD
Associate Clinical Professor
Department of Psychiatry and Human Behavior
University of California, Irvine, College of Medicine

Rhoda K Hahn, MD

Christopher Reist, MD
Associate Professor and Vice Chair
Department of Psychiatry and Human Behavior
University of California, Irvine, College of Medicine

Current Clinical Strategies Publishing
www.ccspublishing.com/ccs

Digital Book and Updates

Purchasers of this book may download the digital book and updates for Palm, Pocket PC, Windows and Macintosh. The digital book can be downloaded at the Current Clinical Strategies Publishing Internet site:

www.ccspublishing.com/ccs/psydrug.htm

Current Clinical Strategies Publishing
PO Box 1753
Blue Jay, CA 92317
Phone: 800-331-8227
Fax: 800-965-9420
Internet: www.ccspublishing.com/ccs

Indications for medications contained in this book sometimes may not be approved by the FDA. Varying degrees of empirical evidence exist for the effectiveness of medications for non- FDA approved uses. The authors have included those off-label indications where sufficient research has been completed to warrant the consideration of these agents as treatment alternatives.

Printed in USA   ISBN 978-1-934323-02-1

Contents

Treatment Adherence

I. Adherence refers to the ability of the patient to comply with the treatment plan to which they have agreed. Assessment of adherence should be done regularly. Problems with treatment adherence arise from 4 primary sources:

   A. **Patient Characteristics:** Attitudes about illness (stigma) as well as towards medications are key determinants of a patient's willingness to accept treatment. Social circumstances, such as the degree of independence or supervision and housing stability, can also affect adherence.

   B. **Clinician Factors:** The ability to develop a good rapport and capacity for empathy is critical for successful treatment. Positive expectancy and competence in pharmacological prescribing and use of non-pharmacological therapies is important.

   C. **Medication Factors:** Many patients have medical and psychiatric comorbidity that result in the need for multiple medications. Adherence is proportional to simplicity. Using medications that are simple, such as once-a-day dosing, can improve adherence. Side effects are also a critical aspect of medication adherence.

   D. **Clinical Features:** Psychiatric disorders are often associated with guilt, paranoia, and anxiety. Cognitive limitations (as a consequence of illness) can be a barrier to gaining insight and remembering to take medications. Substance abuse is often associated with non-adherence.

II. **Evaluation of Treatment Adherence**

   A. Ask patient: Patients who are evasive in response to inquiries about medication effects may be non-adherent. Checking with family or other members of the patients' support system can provide valuable information related to treatment adherence.

   B. Checking prescription refills can verify that the patient is obtaining medication on a consistent schedule.

   C. Missed or chronically rescheduled appointments can be indicative of patient adherence issues.

III. **General Principles for Improving Adherence**

   A. Atypical antipsychotic medications have significantly fewer side effects and should be used as a first line treatment. Depot formulations are available (ex: Risperdal Consta).

   B. A provider should be aware of the patient's understanding of illness as well as attitudes towards medications. Cognitive behavioral therapy and motivational interviewing are useful approaches to negative attitudes or resistance to treatment.

   C. Effective symptom control improves adherence. Symptoms such as paranoia can interfere with patient adherence.

   D. Provide medication education to your patient and their families, either directly or through medication education groups.

   E. Inquire about side effects regularly. If distressing side effects occur, adjust dose, switch medication or treat side effects. More frequent visits during the crossover to the new medication can reduce relapse.

F. Avoid polypharmacy. Multiple medications can significantly increase side effects. Adherence declines as the regimen becomes more complex.

G. Keep treatment regimens simple. Adherence is directly proportional to complexity of medication schedule. Utilize reminder strategies for patients that tend to forget doses.

H. Establish formal procedures to follow-up every missed appointment or no show. Look for ways to reach out to patients who use scheduling conflicts or rescheduling as a way to avoid treatment.

Management of Factors Influencing Adherence	
Factor	Management
Negative drug attitudes	Understand how the patient views medications and illness and address their concerns.
Impaired memory and executive function	Cognitive deficits may interfere with the ability to understand and remember treatment plans. Keep regimens simple and use reminder strategies (alarms, pill box).
Side effects	Regularly ask about side effects and address problematic side effects.
Persisting psychiatric symptoms	Maximize the effectiveness of medication treatment through appropriate dosing.

Antidepressants

Serotonin-Specific Reuptake Inhibitors

I. Indications
- **A.** Serotonin-Specific Reuptake Inhibitors (SSRIs) are the most widely prescribed class of antidepressants. SSRIs have proven efficacy in the treatment of major depression, dysthymia, obsessive-compulsive disorder (OCD), panic disorder, bulimia nervosa, post-traumatic stress disorder, generalized anxiety disorder and social phobia (social anxiety disorder).
- **B.** SSRIs are also effective in the treatment of bipolar depression (but should always be used in conjunction with a mood stabilizer) and premenstrual dysphoric disorder. These agents have some efficacy in the treatment of pain syndromes, such as migraine headaches and chronic pain, but appear to be less effective than tricyclics. There is some evidence that they be effective in impulse control disorders, and the physical/emotional symptoms of menopause.
- **C.** Fluoxetine is approved for use in children for major depressive disorder and OCD. Sertraline is approved for use in children for OCD only.
- **D.** Paroxetine, duloxetine, venlafaxine, and citalopram are not FDA indicated for use in children.

II. Pharmacology
- **A.** SSRIs block serotonin reuptake into presynaptic nerve terminals, leading to enhanced serotonergic neurotransmission.
- **B.** The half-life for most of these agents is approximately 24 hours for the parent compound. Fluoxetine, however, has a half-life of 2-4 days, and the active metabolite of fluoxetine, norfluoxetine, has a 7- to 10-day half-life. Thus, fluoxetine requires over a month to reach steady-state plasma concentrations while the other SSRIs take approximately 5 days.
- **C.** With the exception of escitalopram and fluvoxamine, the SSRIs are highly bound to plasma proteins. SSRIs have significantly less effect on muscarinic, histaminic, and adrenergic receptors, compared to tricyclic antidepressants (TCAs), and the SSRIs are better tolerated.

III. Clinical Guidelines
- **A. Dosage:** SSRIs have the advantage of once-daily dosing. The standard dosage of fluoxetine, citalopram, and paroxetine is 20 mg per day; the dosage should be decreased to 10 mg per day in the elderly. The initial dose of escitalopram is 10 mg/day. Sertraline and fluvoxamine are dosed at 50 mg per day, but the dosage is decreased to 25 mg per day in elderly patients. There is no linear relationship between the SSRI dose and the response. For many patients, the dosage does not need to be increased.
- **B. Obsessive Compulsive Disorder and Bulimia:** Higher dosages of SSRIs, such as 60-80 mg of fluoxetine or 200-300 mg of sertraline, have been used to treat obsessive-compulsive disorder and bulimia. While high doses may be necessary in some patients, many patients will respond to standard dosing after 6-12 weeks. When greater than 40 mg a day of fluoxetine is given, the dosage should be divided into two doses to minimize side effects.

- **C. Panic Disorder:** Patients with panic disorder should be started at a low dosage to prevent increased anxiety in the initial weeks of treatment. Patients should start at 12.5- 25 mg of sertraline, 5-10 mg of paroxetine, 10 mg of citalopram, 5 mg of escitalopram, or 5 mg of fluoxetine. After 1 week, the dosage may be increased gradually to standard dosages.
- **D. Response Time:** SSRIs require 2-4 weeks to begin to alleviate symptoms of depression, and treatment should continue for 6-8 weeks before a patient is considered non-responsive to treatment.
- **E. Plasma Levels:** There is no correlation between plasma concentrations of SSRIs and clinical efficacy. Measuring plasma levels is not clinically indicated.
- **F. Safety:** SSRIs are much safer in overdose than other antidepressants, such as TCAs or MAOIs (monoamine oxidase inhibitors).
- **G. Suicidality:** The FDA has issued a black box warning for the use of all SSRIs in children and adolescents with regard to the increased risk of "suicidal thinking and behavior." The emergence of suicidality is also listed as a risk in adults but not at the level of a black box warning

IV. Adverse Drug Reactions

- **A. Tolerability:** SSRIs are better tolerated than TCAs or MAOIs.
    1. **Alpha-1 Blockade:** SSRIs do not produce orthostatic hypotension because they do not block alpha-1-adrenergic receptors like tricyclic agents.
    2. **Histamine Blockade:** SSRIs produce markedly less sedation or weight gain than TCAs or MAOIs because of minimal effect on histamine receptors.
    3. **Muscarinic Blockade:** SSRIs usually do not cause dry mouth, constipation, blurred vision, or urinary retention because they have minimal effect on muscarinic cholinergic receptors.
    4. **Seizures:** SSRIs have a seizure rate of approximately 0.2%, which is slightly lower than the rate for TCAs.
- **B. Side Effects:** The side effects of SSRIs are primarily mediated by their interaction with serotonergic neurotransmission:
    1. **Gastrointestinal effects,** such as nausea and diarrhea, are the most common adverse reactions. Nausea usually improves after the first few days of treatment. Giving the medication with food often alleviates the nausea.
    2. **Decreased appetite** is common early in treatment because of nausea, and this problem usually improves after several days.
    3. **Headaches** (usually transient) occur occasionally upon initiation of treatment. In some patients, headaches are persistent.
    4. **Insomnia** may occur with any of the SSRIs, but it is more common with fluoxetine and sertraline. Insomnia usually responds to treatment with trazodone 50-100 mg qhs. The SSRI should be given in the morning if insomnia occurs.
    5. SSRIs are less sedating than tricyclic antidepressants, but sedation can occur with paroxetine or fluvoxamine. If sedation occurs, the medication should be given at bedtime.
    6. Sexual dysfunction, such as decreased libido, erectile dysfunction, delayed ejaculation and anorgasmia can occur, and this problem may be treated with Sildenafil (Viagra) 50-100 mg taken one hour before sex, tadalafil (Cialis) 5-20 mg prior to sexual activity, vardenafil (Levitra)

5-20 mg one hour before sex, bupropion (Wellbutrin) 75-150 mg bid, buspirone (BuSpar) 5-20 mg bid-tid, mirtazapine 15-30 mg one hour before sex, nefazodone 100 mg one hour before sex or switching the antidepressant to bupropion, nefazodone or mirtazapine.

7. Serotonin syndrome, characterized by nausea, confusion, hyperthermia, autonomic instability, tremor, myoclonus, rigidity, seizures, coma and death, can occur when SSRIs are combined with MAOIs. SSRIs should not be used for 2 weeks before or after the use of an MAOI. For fluoxetine, 5-6 weeks should elapse after discontinuation of the MAOI because of its long half-life.

C. **Miscellaneous Side Effects:** SSRIs may also cause sweating, anxiety, dizziness, tremors, fatigue, and dry mouth.

D. **Mania:** SSRIs, like all other antidepressants, can induce mania or rapid cycling in bipolar patients. However, the tricyclics are more likely to induce mania than SSRIs.

E. **SSRI Discontinuation Syndrome**: On discontinuation, some patients may experience dizziness, lethargy, nausea, irritability, and headaches. These symptoms are usually transient and are more likely to occur with short-acting agents, such as paroxetine and fluvoxamine. These symptoms can be prevented by slowly tapering the medication over several weeks when discontinuing the drug. Discontinuation of paroxetine may be complicated by cholinergic rebound symptoms, such as diarrhea.

F. **Restlessness:** An akathisia-like syndrome has been reported with fluoxetine. Akathisia can be treated by reducing the dose of the SSRI. Agitation can be profound and often requires discontinuation of the medication.

G. **Teratogenic Effects:** All SSRIs are pregnancy category C. There is no evidence that SSRIs cause major birth defects. A recent FDA advisory (December 2005) suggests a possible link between exposure to paroxetine in the first trimester and an increased risk of cardiac birth defects. The impact of untreated depression on the mother and fetus must be considered when determining these risk-benefit decisions.

H. **Nonteratogenic Effects:** There has been some recent data suggesting a possible risk of persistent pulmonary hypertension (PPHN) in newborns whose mothers took SSRIs or SNRIs after the 20th week of gestation. Less serious difficulties, such as irritability, difficulty feeding requiring some degree of respiratory support have also been described.

I. **Breast Feeding:** SSRIs are secreted into breast milk in minute amounts. A careful discussion of the risk-benefit ratio should occur prior to breastfeeding.

V. **Drug Interactions**

A. **Cytochrome P450 Enzymes:** SSRIs are competitive inhibitors of a variety of cytochrome P450 liver enzymes. This can result in elevated plasma levels of medications metabolized by these enzymes. Elevated plasma levels may lead to toxic side effects.

B. **Potential Toxicity:** Toxic side effects of desipramine can be seen when it is given concomitantly with SSRIs, such as fluoxetine and paroxetine. Desipramine is metabolized by the liver enzyme cytochrome P4502D6 (CYP2D6) and fluoxetine is a potent inhibitor of cytochrome CYP2D6. Fluoxetine can elevate plasma desipramine levels up to 400%, with subsequent increased sedation, anticholinergic effects, tremors and potential increased risk of seizures or cardiotoxicity.

C. Substrates/Inhibitors
1. Table 1 lists the substrates of several P450 liver enzymes, and table 2 indicates the degree of inhibition of the enzymes by each SSRI. The greater the inhibition, the greater the likelihood of a drug-drug interaction.
2. Drugs that have a narrow therapeutic index are more likely to produce toxic symptoms when combined with a strong inhibitor of their metabolism. Drugs with a narrow therapeutic index include antiarrhythmics, anticonvulsants, warfarin, and Theophylline.

D. Warfarin: SSRIs may increase levels of warfarin via P450 interactions and competition for plasma protein binding sites. Prothrombin times should be carefully monitored when initiating SSRIs in a patient on warfarin.

Table 1. Substrates of the P450 Enzymes

CYP1A2	Acetaminophen	Grepafloxen	Pentoxifylline
	Amitriptyline	Haloperidol	Phenacetin
	Caffeine	Imipramine	Propranolol
	Clomipramine	Mexiletine	R-Warfarin
	Clozapine	Mirtazapine	Ropinorole
	Cyclobenzaprine	Methadone	Tacrine
	Dacarbazine	Odansetron	Theophylline
	Flutamide	Olanzapine	Thioridazine
	Fluvoxamine	Paracetamol	Thiothixene
CYP2D6	Amitriptyline	Flecainide	Perphenazine
	Amphetamine	Haloperidol	Propafenone
	Bufaralol	Hydrocodone	Propranolol
	Benztropine	Imipramine	Quinidine
	Clomipramine	MCPP	Quetiapine
	Clozapine	Metoprolol	Risperidone
	Codeine	Mexiletine	Sertraline
	Debrisoquine	Mirtazapine	Sparteine
	Desipramine	Molindone	Tamoxifen
	Dextromethorphan	Nortriptyline	Thioridazine
	Diltiazem	Odansetron	Timolol
	Donepezil	Oxycodone	Trazodone
	Encainide	Paroxetine	Tramadol
	Ethylmorphine	Perhexiline	Venlafaxine
CYP2C9	Carmustine	Losartan	S-Warfarin
	Celecoxib	Mefenamic acid	Suprofen
	Diclofenac	Naproxen	Tamoxifen
	Glyburide	Phenytoin	Tetrahydrocannabinol
	Glypizide	Piroxicam	Tolbutamide
	Ibuprofen	Paclitaxel	Torsemide
	Indomethacin	Rosiglitazone	Valsartan
CYP2C19	Amitriptyline	Imipramine	Pantoprazole
	Citalopram	Lansoprazole	Proguanil
	Clomipramine	Mephobarbital	Propranolol
	Cyclophosphamide	Mephenytoin	Rabeprazole
	Diazepam	Moclobemide	Teniposide
	Hexobarbital	Omeprazole	

12 Serotonin-Specific Reuptake Inhibitors

CYP3A4			
	Acetaminophen	Dirithromycin	Propafenone
	Alfentanil	Disopyramide	Primaquine
	Alprazolam	Donepezil	Progesterone
	Amiodarone	Efavirenz	Quetiapine
	Amitriptyline	Ergots	Quinidine
	Amlodipine	Erythromycin	Rabeprazole
	Amprenavir	Estradiol	Rapamycin
	Avorvastatin	Estrogen	Rifabutin
	Azithromycin	Ethosuximide	Rifampin
	Bromocriptine	Etoposide	Rokitamycin
	Bulsulfan	Felodipine	Ropinirole
	Buspirone	Fentanyl	Saquinous
	Carbamazepine	Imipramine	Sibutramine
	Carvedilol	Indinavir	Sildenafil
	Cerivastatin	Isofamide	Simvastatin
	Chlordiazepoxide	Ketoconazole	Tacrolimus
	Chloroquine	Lansoprazole	Tamoxifen
	Ciprofloxacin	Mirtazapine	Temazepam
	Cilostazol	Lidocaine	Tenoposide
	Cisapride	Lopinavir	Testosterone
	Citalopram	Loratadine	Tiagabine
	Clarithromycin	Lovastatin	Toremifene
	Clomipramine	Metoprolol	Trazodone
	Clonazepam	Midazolam	Triazolam
	Clozapine	Nefazodone	Trofosfamide
	Cortisol	Nevirapine	Troleandomycin
	Cyclobenzaprine	Nicardipine	Valproate
	Cyclosporine	Nifedipine	Verapamil
	Cyclophosphamide	Nimodipine	Vesnarinone
	Dapsone	Nisoldipine	Vinblastine
	Danorubicin	Nitrendipine	Vincristine
	Delavirdine	Odansetron	Vindesine
	Dexamethasone	Omeprazole	Vinorelbine
	Diazepam	Pantoprazole	Zaleplon
	Diltiazem	Paclitaxel	Zolpidem
	Dirithromycin	Pergolide	

Table 2. Degree of Inhibition of Cytochrome P450 Enzymes by SSRIs					
	1A2	**2C9**	**2C19**	**2D6**	**3A4**
Escitalopram (Lexapro)	0/+	0/+	0/+	+	0/+
Citalopram (Celexa)	0/+	0/+	0/+	+	0/+
Fluoxetine (Prozac)	0/+	++/+++	++/+++	++++	+/++
Fluvoxamine (LuVox)	++++	0/+	++++	0/+	+++
Paroxetine (Paxil)	0/+	0/+	0/+	++++	0/+
Sertraline (Zoloft)	0/+	0/+	+/++	+	0/+

Citalopram (Celexa)

I. **Indications:** Effective for a variety of depressive and anxiety disorders.
   Preparations: 10, 20 and 40 mg (20 mg and 40 mg tablets are scored). Oral suspension: 10 mg/5 mL. Generic preparation available.
II. **Dosage:**
   Depression: 20 mg per day, usually given at bedtime. The dosage may be increased to 40 mg per day after one week. Maximum dosage is 60 mg/day, and this dosage should be reserved for treatment refractory patients who have had a 4- to 6-week trial at 40 mg/day.
   Elderly: 10 mg per day for one week, then increase to 20 mg/day. Treatment refractory patients may require 40 mg/day after a trial of 4-6 weeks on 20 mg/day.
III. **Half-Life: 35 hr.**
IV. **Clinical Guidelines:** Citalopram has low overall effects on P450 enzymes (see table 2).
V. **Drug Interactions:** Cytochrome P450: Modest inhibition of the hepatic enzyme, CYP2D6, may lead to mild elevations of TCAs and antiarrhythmics (see Tables 1 & 2). This interaction is unlikely to be clinically significant,

Escitalopram (Lexapro)

I. **Indications:** Effective for a variety of depressive and anxiety disorders.
   Preparations: 5 mg (unscored), 10 and 20 mg scored tablets.
   Oral solution: 5 mg/5 mL.
II. **Dosage:**
   Depression: 10 mg per day. The dosage may be increased to 20 mg per day after one week. Maximum dosage is 30 mg/day, and this dosage should be reserved for treatment refractory patients who have had a 4- to 6-week trial at 20 mg/day.
   Generalized Anxiety Disorder: Same as for depression
   Elderly: 5-10 mg per day. Treatment refractory patients may require 20 mg/day after a trial of 4-6 weeks on 10 mg/day.
III. **Half-Life: 30 hr.**
   A. **Clinical Guidelines:** Compared to the SSRIs, escitalopram has low overall effects on P450 enzymes (see table 2). Compared to the racemate (citalopram), escitalopram has an improved side-effect profile.
   B. **Drug Interactions:** Cytochrome P450: Modest inhibition of the hepatic enzyme, CYP2D6, may lead to mild elevations of TCAs and antiarrhythmics (see Tables 1 & 2). This interaction is unlikely to be clinically significant.

Fluoxetine (Prozac, Sarafem, Prozac Weekly)

I. **Indications:** Effective for depressive and anxiety disorders.
   Preparations: 10, 20 mg capsules; 20 mg/5 mL solution; 10 mg scored tablet; 90 mg weekly tablet. Generic preparation available.
II. **Dosage:**
   A. **Depression:** 20 mg qAM is usually effective. May increase to maximum dose of 80 mg/day. Increase dose by 20 mg/day each month in partial responders. Most patients respond at a dosage between 20-40 mg/day.
   B. **Obsessive-Compulsive Disorder (OCD):** 20 mg/day. Increase by 20 mg/day each month if needed. Treatment of OCD may require a higher dosage than depression. Maximum dose of 80 mg/day.
   C. **Panic Disorder:** Begin with 5-10 mg qAM. Increase gradually over several weeks to 10-20 mg/day.
   D. **Bulimia:** Begin with 20 mg qAM and increase as tolerated up to 60 mg/day over several days to weeks.
   E. **Premenstrual Dysphoric Disorder (PMDD):** Begin with 20 mg/day throughout the month. May be increased up to 60 mg/day.
   F. **Elderly:** 5-40 mg/day. Due to the long half-life, elderly patients require lower doses and every-other-day dosing may be used.
   G. **Half-Life:** 2-5 days for fluoxetine and 7-10 days for the active metabolite of fluoxetine, norfluoxetine.
III. **Clinical Guidelines**
   A. Long half-life permits daily dosing and decrease withdrawal symptoms following abrupt discontinuance of medication. Relatively safe in over-dose.

B. The long half-life of fluoxetine/norfluoxetine requires waiting at least 5 weeks after discontinuation before starting an MAOI. Several weeks should elapse before beginning nefazodone, because the metabolite of nefazodone may cause anxiety, and the metabolism of nefazodone is impaired by fluoxetine. Patients often require bid dosing above 40 mg per day. Typical dosing is 40 mg in the morning and 20-40 mg at noon. Late afternoon doses often disrupt sleep.

IV. Drug Interactions

   A. Fluoxetine is a potent inhibitor of the liver enzyme, cytochrome CYP2D6. Use caution when combining with a TCA or an antiarrhythmic agent. Can also elevate levels of many neuroleptic agents, leading to dystonias, akathisia, or other extrapyramidal symptoms.

   B. Benzodiazepines: Inhibition of the liver enzyme, CYP3A4, can lead to moderate plasma elevations of some benzodiazepines with increased sedation and psychomotor impairment.

   C. Carbamazepine: Inhibition of the liver enzyme, CYP3A4, can elevate carbamazepine levels moderately. Carbamazepine levels should be monitored.

   D. Phenytoin: Modest elevations of phenytoin occur because of inhibition of the liver enzyme, CYP2C9. Phenytoin levels should be monitored.

   E. Opiate Analgesics: Patients taking fluoxetine will experience reduced pain relief from codeine, hydrocodone and oxycodone. CYP2D6 inhibition will reduce conversion of the parent analgesic to the clinically effective metabolite.

   F. Fluoxetine has slightly higher rates of anxiety and insomnia than the other SSRIs.

   G. Refer to tables 1 and 2 for other potential drug interactions.

Fluvoxamine (Luvox)

I. Indications: Effective for a variety of depressive and anxiety disorders.
   Preparations: 25, 50, 100 mg tablets (50 and 100 mg tablets are scored). Generic preparation available.

II. Dosage:
   Initial Dosage: 50 mg/day, then titrate to 300 mg/day maximum, over several weeks
   Elderly: 25-150 mg/day
   Children: 25 mg/day initially, then increase by 25 mg/week as needed to 50-200 mg/day

III. Half-Life: 16-20 hours.

IV. Clinical Guidelines: Patients often require bid dosing at dosages above 100-200 mg per day. Many drug interactions with cytochrome P450 metabolized medications have been reported. Since other SSRIs are equally effective, it is not commonly used.

V. Drug Interactions

   A. Theophylline: Potent inhibition of the hepatic enzyme, CYP1A2, can produce toxicity in combination with theophylline, resulting in elevated plasma levels of other CYP1A2 substrates.

   B. Clozapine: Potent inhibition of CYP1A2 can lead to markedly elevated clozapine levels with potential for seizures and hypotension. Olanzapine levels will also be increased.

C. Benzodiazepines: Significant inhibition of the hepatic enzyme, CYP3A4, can lead to elevated levels of some benzodiazepines, such as alprazolam, with subsequent increased sedation and psychomotor impairment.

D. Beta-Blockers: Significant inhibition of the hepatic enzyme, CYP2C19, can lead to elevated plasma concentrations of propranolol, with further reductions in heart rate and hypotension.

E. Calcium Channel Blockers: Inhibition of the hepatic enzyme, CYP3A4, can produce elevated levels of calcium channel blockers, such as diltiazem, with subsequent bradycardia.

F. Methadone: Fluvoxamine can significantly raise plasma methadone levels.

G. Carbamazepine: Fluvoxamine may elevate carbamazepine levels via CYP3A4 inhibition, leading to toxicity.

H. Refer to tables 1 and 2 for other potential drug interactions.

Paroxetine (Paxil, Paxil CR)

I. Indications: Effective for a variety of depressive and anxiety disorders.
Preparations: 10, 20, 30, 40 mg tablets (10 and 20 mg tablets are scored); 10 mg/5 mL oral solution; 12.5, 25, and 37.5 mg continuous-release formulation. Generic preparation available.

II. Dosage:
A. Depression: 10-20 mg qhs; may increase dose by 10-20 mg/day each month if partial response occurs (maximum 80 mg/day). For Paxil CR, begin at 25 mg/day and adjust upwards by 12.5 mg per week if needed to a maximum dosage of 62.5 mg/day.

B. Obsessive-Compulsive Disorder: 20 mg per day to start, then increase by 10-20 mg/day per month if partial response occurs (maximum 80 mg/day).

C. Panic Disorder: Begin with 5-10 mg qhs, then increase dose by 10 mg every 2-4 weeks as tolerated until symptoms abate, up to 40 mg/day. For Paxil CR, begin at 12.5 mg/day and increase by 12.5 mg per week as needed up to a maximum dosage of 75 mg per day.

D. Social Anxiety Disorder: Begin with 20 mg qhs. In highly anxious patients, an initial dosage of 10 mg qhs for one week, then 20 mg qhs, may reduce side effects. If clinical response is inadequate, increase the dosage by 10-20 mg/every 4-6 weeks to a maximum dosage of 60 mg/day.

E. Elderly: 5-40 mg/day for immediate release and 12.5 to 50 mg per day for Paxil CR.

III. Half-Life: 15-20 hours

IV. Clinical Guidelines: A reduction in anxiety often occurs early in treatment due to sedating properties. Paroxetine is less activating than fluoxetine and more sedating than fluoxetine or sertraline for most patients. Paroxetine should be taken at bedtime because it has sedative properties compared to fluoxetine or sertraline. Relatively safe in overdose. Patients may require bid dosing at dosages above 40 mg per day. Paxil CR at a dosage of 37.5 mg is bioequivalent to 30 mg of immediate-release Paxil. Paxil CR may have less

side effects compared to immediate-release paroxetine.
V. Drug Interactions
   A. Paroxetine is a potent inhibitor of the liver enzyme, CYP2D6. Use caution when combining with TCAs or antiarrhythmics. Can also elevate levels of some neuroleptics and increase the incidence of EPS. Refer to tables 1 and 2 for additional potential drug interactions.
   B. Patients on paroxetine will experience reduced pain relief from codeine, hydrocodone and oxycodone. CYP2D6 inhibition will reduce conversion of the parent analgesic to the clinically effective metabolite of the analgesic.
   C. Paroxetine produces the highest incidence of discontinuation syndrome of the SSRIs because its relatively short half-life and anticholinergic activity, complicating the discontinuation syndrome with cholinergic rebound.
II. Recent evidence has linked paroxetine use in the first trimester and increased risk of cardiac birth defects.

Sertraline (Zoloft)

I. Indications: Effective for a variety of depressive and anxiety disorders.
   Preparations: 25, 50, 100 mg scored tablets; 20 mg/mL oral suspension. Generic preparation available.
II. Dosage:
   A. **Depression:** 50 mg qAM, then increase by 50 mg/day every month in patients with partial response (maximum dose of 200 mg/day).
   B. **Obsessive-Compulsive Disorder:** Begin with 50 mg qAM and increase by 50 mg/day per month in partial responders to a maximum of 200-300 mg/day.
   C. **Panic Disorder/Post-Traumatic Stress Disorder:** Begin with 25 mg qAM and increase dose by 25 mg/day every 2-4 weeks until symptoms abate, to a maximum dose of 200 mg/day. Patients with severe anxiety or sensitivity to medication may be started at 12.5 mg for the first week.
   D. **Elderly:** 25-150 mg/day.
   E. **Premenstrual Dysphoric Disorder (PMDD):** 50 mg per day throughout the menstrual cycle or limited to the luteal phase.
   F. **Children:** 25 mg/day for ages 6-12 and 50 mg/day for adolescents age 13-17.
III. Half-Life: 24 hours for sertraline and 2-4 days for its metabolite, desmethyl-sertraline.
IV. Clinical Guidelines: Sertraline is less likely to cause sedation compared to paroxetine or fluvoxamine. Restlessness and insomnia are less common compared to fluoxetine. Sertraline, escitalopram and citalopram have the lowest overall P450 enzyme effects of the SSRIs (refer to table 2).
V. Drug Interactions: Cytochrome P450: Modest inhibition of the hepatic enzyme, CYP2D6, may lead to mild elevations of TCAs and antiarrhythmics.

References, see page 115.

Miscellaneous Antidepressants

The following antidepressants are unique compounds that are chemically unrelated to the SSRIs, TCAs and MAOIs. They are indicated for depression and require the same amount of time to achieve clinical efficacy. Like other antidepressants, these agents may cause mania or rapid cycling in bipolar patients. The use of MAOIs with these antidepressants can lead to a sero-tonergic syndrome, characterized by nausea, confusion, hyperthermia, autonomic instability, tremor, myoclonus, rigidity, seizures, coma and death. These antidepressants are contraindicated for two weeks before or after the use of an MAOI.

Bupropion (Wellbutrin, Wellbutrin SR, Wellbutrin XL, Zyban)

I. **Indications**
   A. Bupropion is effective in the treatment of major depression, dysthymia, and bipolar depression. Bupropion is also used for the treatment of Attention-Deficit Hyperactivity Disorder.
   B. Low-dose bupropion is used adjunctively to treat the sexual dysfunction associated with SSRIs.

II. **Pharmacology**
   A. Bupropion is a unicyclic aminoketone antidepressant with a half-life of 4-24 hours. It is thought to work via inhibition of norepinephrine reuptake and by inhibition of dopaminegic neurotransmission.
   B. Therapeutic levels have not been established.

III. **Clinical Guidelines**
   A. Preparations: 75 and 100 mg immediate-release tablets; 100, 150 and 200 mg sustained-release tablets, 150 and 300 mg extended-release tablets. All tablets are non-scored. Generic preparation available.
   B. **Dosage**
      1. **Initial Dosage:** 100 mg bid, then increase to 100 tid after 4-5 days. Although bupropion has a short half-life and is recommended for tid dosing, many clinicians use bid dosing with the regular-release tablets as well as the sustained release. Do not increase by more than 100/day mg every 3 days.
      2. **Slow Release:** Begin with 150 mg qAM for three days, then increase to 150 mg bid for SR tabs. Maximum dose of 200 mg SR tabs bid. The sustained-release bid preparation improves compliance.
      3. **Average Dosage:** 300 mg/day (divided doses). Do not exceed 150 mg/dose for the regular release or 200 mg/dose with sustained release, with doses at least 6 hours apart.
      4. **Dosage Range:** 75-450 mg/day (max 450 mg/day).
      5. **Elderly:** 75-450 mg/day.
   C. **Side-Effect Profile:** Bupropion has fewer side effects than TCAs and

causes less sexual dysfunction than the SSRIs. It does not produce weight gain or orthostatic hypotension.

D. Cardiac Profile: Bupropion does not significantly affect cardiac conduction or ventricular function and is a good choice in patients with cardiac disease, such as congestive heart failure.

IV. Adverse Drug Reactions

A. Most common side effects: Insomnia, CNS stimulation, headache, constipation, dry mouth, nausea, tremor.

B. Anorexia/Bulimia: Avoid bupropion in patients with anorexia or bulimia because of possible electrolyte changes, which may potentiate seizures.

C. Liver/Renal Disease: Use caution in patients with hepatic or renal disease because of potential elevation of plasma bupropion levels and toxicity.

D. Pregnancy/Lactation: Recent change to Pregnancy category C based on studies in rabbits.

E. Seizures: Bupropion has a seizure rate of 0.4% at doses less than 450 mg/day and 4% at doses of 450-600 mg/day. The sustained-release preparation has a seizure incidence of 0.1% at doses up to 300 mg per day. Bupropion is contraindicated in patients with a history of seizure, brain injury or EEG abnormality, or recent history of alcohol withdrawal.

V. Drug Interactions

A. Hepatically Metabolized Medications

1. Cimetidine may inhibit the metabolism of bupropion and lead to elevated bupropion plasma levels and subsequent toxicity.

2. Bupropion is a significant inhibitor of **CYP2D6** and can cause a twofold increase in maximum concentration or fivefold increase in area under the plasma concentration curve (AUC) of CYP2D6 substrates, such as desipramine. If bupropion is added to a treatment regimen of medications metabolized by CYP2D6, the dosage of the other medications may need to be reduced. Medications metabolized by CYP2D6 include tricyclic antidepressants, type 1C antiarrhythmics and beta-blockers (such as Metoprolol).

3. **Carbamazepine, phenobarbital, and phenytoin** may induce the enzymes responsible for the metabolism of bupropion, resulting in a subsequent decrease in plasma bupropion levels.

4. **Dopamine Agonists:** Levodopa may cause confusion or dyskinesias.

B. MAOIs: Combining bupropion with an MAOI can lead to a serotonergic syndrome with severe toxicity.

Duloxetine (Cymbalta)

I. Indications
A. Duloxetine is effective for the treatment of major depression. It is helpful for somatization disorders and pain syndromes associated with depression.

B. Cymbalta is a new medication with limited clinical experience to date.

II. Pharmacology
A. Duloxetine blocks serotonin and norepinephrine reuptake.

B. Half-life is 12 hours.

III. Clinical Guidelines
A. Preparations: 20, 30 and 60 mg capsules.

    1. Dosage

        a. Initial dosage: 20 mg po bid, may increase to 30 mg bid.

        b. Average dosage: 30 mg bid. Doses as high as 60 mg bid may be preferred for the treatment of pain syndromes.

    2. No dosage adjustment is necessary in healthy geriatric patients.

    3. A discontinuation syndrome can be observed with abrupt cessation of treatment.

IV. Adverse Drug Reactions
A. Common Adverse Reactions: Nausea (most common), decreased appetite, dry mouth, dizziness, constipation, fatigue, sweating and insomnia. There is a small incidence of sexual dysfunction, primarily in men.

B. Cymbalta may cause elevated liver enzymes, hepatitis, and cholestatic jaundice. These effects are more likely in patients with substantial alcohol use or pre-existing liver disease.

V. Drug Interactions:
Duloxetine is metabolized through CYP2D6 and 1A2. Inhibition of these enzymes will increase serum duloxetine levels.

Gepirone ER

I. Indications (FDA approval pending)
A. Gepirone is effective in the treatment of major depression.

II. Pharmacology
A. Gepirone is a pyridinyl piperazine 5HT1A agonist.

B. Gepirone has differential action at presynaptic (agonist) and post-synaptic (partial agonist) 5-HT1A receptors. Compared to buspirone, it has much less D2 receptor affinity.

III. Clinical Guidelines
A. Preparations: Extended-release 20 mg tablets.

B. Dosage

    1. Initial dosage: 20 mg po qAM, increase every 4 days by 20 mg.

    2. Average dosage: 60 mg/day is likely to be the most common dosage.

    3. Dosage range: 40-80 mg/day.

C. Gepirone has minimal effects on weight, sexual function, or sedation.

IV. Adverse Drug Reactions
A. Common Adverse Reactions: Dizziness, nausea, insomnia, nervousness, dry mouth, and GI distress.

V. Drug Interactions
A. Gepirone does not inhibit P450 enzymes to a significant extent.
B. Because it is metabolized through by the CYP3A4 enzyme (CYP2D6 to a lesser extent) inhibitors of CYP3A4 can alter kinetics.

Mirtazapine (Remeron)

I. **Indications:** Depressive disorders.
II. **Mechanism:** Selective alpha-2-adrenergic antagonist that enhances noradrenergic and serotonergic neurotransmission.
III. **Preparations:** 15 and 30 mg scored tablets.
IV. **Soltabs:** Orally disintegrating tablets (15, 30 and 45 mg).
V. **Dosage**
   A. **Initial Dosage:** Begin with 15 mg qhs and increase to 30 mg after several days to a maximum of 45 mg qhs.
   B. **Elderly:** Begin with 7.5 mg qhs, and increase by 7.5 mg each week to an average of 30 mg qhs.
   C. **Half-Life:** 20-40 hr.
VI. **Therapeutic levels:** Not established.
VII. **Clinical Guidelines**
   A. Mirtazapine has little effect on sexual function. It may have some efficacy in anxiety disorders, and its antagonism of 5-HT3 receptors may help in patients with gastritis. It has little effect on drugs metabolized by cytochrome P450 enzymes.
   B. Sedation is the most common side effect, which may be significant initially, but usually decreases over the first week of treatment.
   C. Increase in appetite is frequent with an average weight gain of 2.0 kg after six weeks of treatment. Dry mouth, constipation, fatigue, dizziness, and orthostatic hypotension may occur.
   D. Agranulocytosis has occurred in two patients, and neutropenia has occurred in one patient during clinical trials with 2,800 patients. If a patient develops signs of an infection along with a low WBC, mirtazapine should be discontinued.
II. **Drug Interactions:** Mirtazapine has a low liability for drug interactions.

Nefazodone (Serzone)

I. **Indications**
   A. Nefazodone is effective in the treatment of major depression, dysthymia, and the depressed phase of bipolar disorder.
   B. Nefazodone is also used clinically for premenstrual dysphoric disorder, chronic pain, and posttraumatic stress disorder.
II. **Pharmacology**
   A. Nefazodone is the phenylpiperazine analog of trazodone and has a half-life of 2-18 hours. Nefazodone inhibits presynaptic serotonin reuptake and blocks postsynaptic serotonin receptors (5HT-2A).
   B. Therapeutic levels have not been established.

III. Clinical Guidelines

A. Preparations: 50, 100, 150, 200, and 250 mg tablets; the 100 and 150 mg tablets are scored.

B. Dosage

1. **Initial dosage:** 50-100 mg bid, then increase gradually over several days to weeks by 50-100 mg per day.
2. **Average dosage:** 300-500 mg/day with bid dosing.
3. **Dosage range:** 50-600 mg/day.
4. **Elderly:** Start with 50 mg/day, range: 100-200 bid.

C. REM Sleep: Nefazodone does not suppress REM sleep, unlike most antidepressants.

D. Sexual Functioning: Nefazodone has no adverse effects on sexual functioning unlike other antidepressants.

IV. Adverse Drug Reactions

A. Common Adverse Reactions: The most common side effects are nausea, dry mouth, dizziness, sedation, agitation, constipation, weight loss, and headaches.

B. Hepatic Disease: Cases of life-threatening hepatic failure have been reported at a rate of 1 case of hepatic failure resulting in death or liver transplant per 250,000-300,000 patient years of nefazodone treatment. Nefazodone should not be initiated if active liver disease or elevated transaminases are present. Patients who develop increased transaminases more than three times normal should discontinue treatment.

C. Alpha-Adrenergic Blockade: Nefazodone produces less orthostatic hypotension than trazodone or tricyclic antidepressants.

D. Histaminic Blockade: Nefazodone has little effect on histamine receptors and produces less weight gain than TCAs or trazodone.

E. Cardiac Effects: Nefazodone does not alter cardiac conduction.

V. Drug Interactions

A. CYP3A4: Nefazodone is a significant inhibitor of the hepatic CYP3A4 enzyme, and levels of all medications metabolized by this enzyme may be elevated. Levels of triazolam and alprazolam may be increased.

B. Cytochrome P450 Inhibitors: A metabolite of nefazodone, chlorophenyl-piperazine (m-CPP), is rapidly inactivated by the cytochrome P450 enzyme system. In the presence of a strong inhibitor of the hepatic CYP2D6 enzyme, such as fluoxetine, m-CPP is not broken down, resulting in anxiety. When switching from fluoxetine or paroxetine to nefazodone, a washout period of 3-4 days for paroxetine and several weeks for fluoxetine is recommended to avoid this adverse reaction.

C. Other Cytochrome P450 Enzymes: Nefazodone does not appear to affect the metabolism of medications metabolized by other P450 enzymes.

D. Digoxin: Nefazodone can produce modest increases in digoxin levels.

E. MAOI: The combination of nefazodone with an MAOI can lead to a serotonergic syndrome and severe toxicity.

Trazodone (Desyrel)

I. Indications
A. Approved for use in depressive disorders. It is also used clinically to reduce anxiety and decrease agitation and aggression in elderly demented patients.

B. Trazodone is commonly prescribed for insomnia, and it is also effective in some patients with chronic pain syndromes.

II. Pharmacology
A. Trazodone is a triazolopyridine with a half-life of 4-9 hours.

B. The efficacy of trazodone is related primarily to inhibition of presynaptic serotonin reuptake, with possible mild postsynaptic serotonergic antagonism.

C. Plasma levels are not clinically useful.

III. Clinical Guidelines
A. **Preparations:** 50, 100, 150, and 300 mg tablets.

B. **Dosage:**
1. **Initial dosage:** 50-100 mg qhs, then increase by 50 mg/day as tolerated. May require bid dosing initially.
2. **Average dosage:** 300-600 mg/day.
3. **Dosage range:** 200-600 mg/day.
4. **Elderly:** 50-500 mg/day.
5. **Insomnia:** 25-200 mg qhs.

C. **Tolerability:** Many patients are unable to tolerate the sedation and hypotension, which significantly limits the utility of trazodone in the treatment of depression. It is, therefore, most often used for insomnia, especially in patients with SSRI-induced insomnia.

IV. Adverse Drug Reactions
A. **Histaminic Blockade:** Trazodone is a potent antihistamine, which can cause significant sedation and weight gain.

B. **Alpha-1-adrenergic Blockade:** Marked Inhibition of alpha-1-adrenergic receptors often leads to severe hypotension, especially at high doses. Reflex tachycardia and dizziness may also occur.

C. **Cholinergic Blockade:** Trazodone has little effect on muscarinic receptors, and it does not produce the anticholinergic effects seen with TCAs.

D. **Dry Mouth**: Trazodone commonly causes dry mouth.

E. **Cardiac Effects:** Trazodone has little effect on cardiac conduction; however, there have been reports of exacerbation of arrhythmias in patients with preexisting conduction abnormalities. It should be avoided in patients with recent myocardial infarction.

F. **Priapism:** A prolonged, painful penile erection occurs in 1/6000 patients. Patients can be treated with intracavernal injection of epinephrine.

G. **Miscellaneous:** Nausea, GI irritation and headaches may occur.

H. **Pregnancy/Lactation:** Avoid use in pregnancy due to potential teratogenicity. Patients should not breast feed while using trazodone.

I. **Overdose:** Trazodone is much safer in overdose than TCAs, but fatalities can occur with combined overdose with alcohol or sedative/hypnotics.

J. **ECT:** Use of trazodone is not recommended during ECT.

V. Drug Interactions

A. **CNS Depressants:** Trazodone may potentiate the effects of other sedating medications.

B. **Fluoxetine** may elevate trazodone levels, but the combination is generally safe, and low-dose trazodone is very effective in treating insomnia due to fluoxetine.

C. **Digoxin/Phenytoin:** Trazodone may elevate plasma levels of these drugs.

D. **Warfarin:** Trazodone has been reported to alter prothrombin time in patients on warfarin.

E. **MAOIs:** Avoid combining trazodone with MAOIs due to the potential of inducing a serotonergic syndrome.

Venlafaxine (Effexor and Effexor XR)

I. Indications

A. Venlafaxine is effective in the treatment of major depression, dysthymia, other depressive disorders and anxiety disorders, such as generalized anxiety disorder.

B. It may have some efficacy in Attention-Deficit Hyperactivity Disorder as well as chronic pain management.

II. Pharmacology

A. Venlafaxine is a phenylethylamine. The half-life is 5 hours for venlafaxine and 10 hours for its active metabolite, O-desmethylvenlafaxine.

B. Venlafaxine is a selective inhibitor of norepinephrine and serotonin reuptake.

C. Therapeutic plasma levels have not been established.

III. Clinical Guidelines

A. **Preparations:** 25, 37.5, 50, 75, 100 mg scored immediate-release tablets; and 37.5, 75, and 150 mg extended-release capsules.

B. **Dosage**

1. **Immediate Release:** 75 mg on the first day in two- or three-divided doses with food. The dose may be increased upward in increments of 75 mg/day as clinically indicated with an average dose between 75 to 225 mg per day in bid dosing. Patients usually require several days before the dosage can be increased.

2. **Extended Release:** Begin with 37.5 to 75 mg once a day with food, and increase the dosage gradually up to 225 mg if needed with an average dosage of 150 to 175 mg per day.

3. **Dosage range:** 75-375 mg/day.

4. **Elderly:** 75-375 mg/day.

5. **Generalized Anxiety Disorder:** Begin with 75 mg q day of Effexor XR; some patients may need to begin with 37.5 mg q day of Effexor XR for one week and then increase to 75 mg q day. The dosage should then be titrated up as clinically indicated to a maximum dosage of 300 mg/day.

IV. Adverse Drug Reactions

A. **Common Side Effects:** Insomnia and anxiety are the most common side effects of venlafaxine. Nausea, sedation, fatigue, sweating, dizziness, headache, loss of appetite, constipation and dry mouth are also common. Some patients have difficulty tolerating the GI distress and sedation.

B. **Blood Pressure:** Elevations of supine diastolic blood pressure to greater than 90 mm Hg and by more than 10 mm Hg above baseline occur in 3-7% of patients. Blood pressure should be monitored periodically in patients on venlafaxine. Blood pressure effects were thought to be limited to the use of immediate-release Effexor, but there are recent case reports of increased blood pressure with XR.

C. **Sexual:** Abnormalities of ejaculation/orgasm occur in approximately 10% of patients.

D. **Seizures:** Seizures occur in 0.3% of patients.

E. **Discontinuation Syndrome:** Venlafaxine has a high incidence of discontinuation syndrome due to its short half-life, and it should not be abruptly discontinued. Venlafaxine can produce dizziness, insomnia, dry mouth, nausea, nervousness, and sweating with abrupt discontinuation. It should be slowly tapered over several weeks when possible.

F. **Renal/Hepatic Disease:** The clearance of venlafaxine in patients with liver or renal disease is significantly altered, and the dosage should be decreased by 50% in these patients.

G. **Cardiac Disease:** There is no systematic data on the use of venlafaxine in patients with recent MI or cardiac disease. It does not appear to have a significant effect on patients with normal cardiac conduction.

H. **Pregnancy/Lactation:** Avoid use in pregnant patients due to potential teratogenic effects. Breast feeding is contraindicated.

V. **Drug Interactions**

A. **Cytochrome P450 Interactions:** Venlafaxine does not appear to cause clinically significant inhibition of hepatic metabolism. It consequently should not significantly inhibit the metabolism of medications metabolized by these enzymes.

B. **MAOIs:** Venlafaxine should not be given concomitantly with an MAOI because of the possibility of producing a serotonergic syndrome with toxicity.

References, see page 115.

Heterocyclic Antidepressants

Tertiary Amine Tricyclic Antidepressants

I. Indications
   A. The heterocyclic antidepressants are used in the treatment of major depression, dysthymia, and the depressed phase of bipolar disorder.
   B. They have efficacy in anxiety disorders, such as panic disorder, social phobia, generalized anxiety disorder, and obsessive-compulsive disorder.
   C. They are useful adjuncts in the treatment of bulimia and chronic pain syndromes.

II. Pharmacology
   A. The heterocyclic antidepressants are postulated to work through their effects on monoamine neurotransmitters, such as serotonin, norepinephrine and dopamine. These agents block the reuptake of these neurotransmitters to varying degrees and also interact with muscarinic, cholinergic, alpha-1-adrenergic, and histaminic receptors, which results in their characteristic side-effect profile.
   B. These antidepressants are rapidly absorbed from the gut and undergo significant first pass clearance by the liver. There is marked variability in plasma levels among individuals, which correlates with differences in cytochrome P450 isoenzymes.
   C. These medications are highly protein bound and lipid soluble. Their half-lives are usually greater than 24 hours, which allows for once-a-day dosing. Steady-state levels are reached in approximately five days.
   D. The tertiary tricyclic antidepressant amines, such as amitriptyline and imipramine, are demethylated to secondary amine metabolites, nortriptyline and desipramine, respectively. The tertiary tricyclic amines have more side effects and greater lethality in overdose because of greater blockade of cholinergic, adrenergic and histaminic receptors compared to secondary amines.

III. Clinical Guidelines
   A. Choice of Drug: The selection of a heterocyclic antidepressant should be based on a patient's past response to medication, family history of medication response, and side-effect profile. For example, if a patient has previously been effectively treated with nortriptyline, there is a good chance of a positive response if the same symptoms recur. Additionally, if a patient is sensitive to the sedative properties of medications, a secondary amine should be chosen over a tertiary amine.
   B. Dosage:
   1. The dosage of heterocyclic antidepressants should be titrated upward over several days to weeks to allow patients to adjust to side effects. This is a major disadvantage compared to SSRIs because it significantly increases the time to reach therapeutic effect in most patients. Most heterocyclics are started at a dose of 25-50 mg per day, and the daily dose is gradually increased to an average of 150-300 mg per day.
   2. Patients with anxiety disorders, such as panic disorder, should receive a lower initial dosage, such as 10 mg of imipramine. Patients with

anxiety disorders may require slow titration to avoid exacerbation of anxiety symptoms.

C. **Time to Response:** A therapeutic trial of at least 3-4 weeks at the maximum tolerated dosage should be completed before a patient is considered a nonresponder. Some patients may require 6-8 weeks of treatment before responding.

IV. **Adverse Drug Reactions**

A. **Elderly patients** are much more sensitive to the side effects of TCAs, and they may be unable to tolerate therapeutic dosages.

B. **Anticholinergic Effects:** Cholinergic blockade can produce dry mouth, blurred vision, constipation, urinary retention, heat intolerance, tachycardia, and exacerbation of narrow angle glaucoma. Constipation may be alleviated by stool softeners. Dry mouth can be improved with the use of sugarless candy.

C. **Alpha-Adrenergic Effects:** Alpha-1-adrenergic receptor blockade can lead to orthostatic hypotension, resulting in falls. Dizziness and reflex tachycardia may also occur.

D. **Histaminic Effects:** Histaminic blockade can produce sedation and weight gain. Many of these agents should be given at bedtime to prevent excess daytime sedation.

E. **Cardiotoxicity**
   1. Heterocyclic antidepressants slow cardiac conduction, leading to intraventricular conduction delays, prolonged PR and QT intervals, AV block, and T-wave flattening.
   2. These agents are contraindicated in patients with pre-existing conduction delays, such as a bundle branch block, or in patients with arrhythmias or recent myocardial infarction. These effects can also be seen with overdose. These agents can also cause tachycardia and elevations of blood pressure.

F. **Seizures:** Seizures occur at a rate of approximately 0.3%, and they are more likely to occur with elevated blood plasma levels, especially with clomipramine, amoxapine, and maprotiline.

G. **Neurotoxicity:** Heterocyclics may produce tremors and ataxia. In overdose, agitation, delirium, seizures, coma and death may occur.

H. **Serotonergic Effects:** Erectile and ejaculatory dysfunction may occur in males, and anorgasmia may occur in females.

I. **Overdose:** Heterocyclic agents are extremely toxic in overdose. Overdose with as little as 1-2 grams may cause death. Death usually occurs from cardiac arrhythmias, seizures, or severe hypotension.

J. **Mania:** Heterocyclic antidepressants can precipitate mania or rapid cycling in patients with bipolar disorder and should only be used in conjunction with a mood stabilizer.

K. **Liver/Renal Disease:** Patients with hepatic or renal disease may require a lower dosage. Severe disease is a contraindication for TCAs.

L. **Discontinuation Syndrome:** Abrupt discontinuation of these agents may lead to transient dizziness, nausea, headache, diaphoresis, insomnia, and malaise. These effects are mostly related to cholinergic and serotonergic rebound. Heterocyclic agents should be tapered gradually over several weeks after prolonged treatment.

M. **Teratogenic Effects:** Heterocyclic antidepressants are classified as pregnancy class C. However, there is no evidence that TCAs cause major

birth defects in humans.
  N. Breast Feeding: Heterocyclics are excreted in breast milk, and mothers should not breast feed when taking these agents.
V. Drug Interactions
  A. Plasma Level Increases: Some of the SSRIs, such as fluoxetine and paroxetine, can elevate heterocyclic antidepressants levels, leading to marked toxicity.
  B. Plasma Level Decreases: Oral contraceptives, carbamazepine, barbiturates, chloral hydrate, and cigarette smoking can induce hepatic enzymes and may lead to decreased levels of heterocyclics.
  C. Antihypertensives: Heterocyclic agents can block the effects of antihypertensive agents such as clonidine and propranolol.
  D. MAOIs: The combination of heterocyclic agents with (MAOIs) can lead to a hypertensive crisis or a "serotonin syndrome," characterized by confusion, agitation, myoclonus, hyperreflexia, autonomic instability, delirium, coma, and even death. MAOIs should be discontinued for 2 weeks before or after the use of a heterocyclic antidepressant.
  E. Anticholinergic Toxicity: The combination of heterocyclics with other medications with anticholinergic properties can potentiate anticholinergic effects and may lead to delirium.

Amitriptyline (Elavil, Endep)

Indications: Depressive disorders, anxiety disorders, chronic pain, and insomnia.
Preparations: 10, 25, 50, 75, 100, 150 mg tablets; 10 mg/mL solution for IM injection.
Dosage
  Initial dosage: 25 mg qhs, then increase over 1- to 4-week period.
  Average dosage: 150-250 mg/day.
  Dosage range: 50-300 mg/day.
  Chronic Pain Syndromes: 25-300 mg qhs.
  Elderly: 25-200 mg/day.
Half-life: 10-50 hr.
Therapeutic Level: 100-250 ng/mL (amitriptyline + nortriptyline).
Clinical Guidelines: Amitriptyline is widely used in the treatment of chronic pain and is effective in the prophylaxis of migraine headaches. Strong anticholinergic effects are often difficult for patients to tolerate. It is useful for insomnia, at a dosage of 25-100 mg qhs.

Clomipramine (Anafranil)

Indications: Depressive disorders and obsessive-compulsive disorder.
Preparations: 25, 50, 75 mg capsules.
Dosage:
  Initial dosage: 25 mg qhs, then increase over 1- to 4-week period.
  Average dose: 150-250 mg/day.
  Dosage Range: 50-250 mg/day.

Panic disorder: 25-150 mg qhs.
Half-life: 20-50 hr.
Therapeutic Level: 150-300 ng/mL
Clinical Guidelines: FDA approved for the treatment of OCD. OCD symptoms may require a longer duration of treatment (2-3 months) to achieve efficacy. Clomipramine may be especially useful in depressed patients with strong obsessional features. The side-effect profile (sedation and anticholinergic effects) often prevents patients from achieving an adequate dosage. Clomipramine has a higher risk of seizures than other TCAs.

Doxepin (Adapin, Sinequan)

Indications: Depressive disorders, anxiety disorders, insomnia, and chronic pain.
Preparations: 15, 25, 50, 75, 100, 150 mg tablets; 10 mg/mL liquid concentrate.
Dosage:
  Initial dosage: 25 mg qhs or bid, then increase over 1- to 4-week period
  Average dosage: 150-250 mg/day.
  Dosage range: 25-300 mg/day.
  Elderly: 15-200 mg/day.
  Insomnia: 25-150 mg qhs.
Half-Life: 8-24 hr.
Therapeutic Levels: 100-250 ng/mL.
Clinical Guidelines: Doxepin may be used in the treatment of chronic pain. It is one of the most sedating TCAs. The strong antihistamine properties of doxepin make it one of the most effective antipruritic agents available. It is useful for insomnia at a dosage of 25-150 mg qhs.

Imipramine (Tofranil)

Indications: Depressive disorders, anxiety disorders, enuresis, chronic pain.
Preparations: 10, 25, 50 mg tablets; 75, 100, 125, 150 mg capsules; 25 mg/2 mL solution for IM injection.
Dosage:
  Initial dosage: 25 mg qhs, then increase over 1- to 4-week period.
  Average dosage: 150-250 mg/day.
  Dosage range: 50-300 mg/day.
  Elderly: 25-75 mg qhs (max 200 mg/day).
Half-Life: 5-25 hr.
Therapeutic Levels: 150-300 ng/mL (imipramine and desipramine)
Clinical Guidelines: Imipramine has well-documented effectiveness in the treatment of panic disorder. Imipramine is effective in the treatment of enuresis in children. The dosage for enuresis is usually 50-100 mg per day.

Trimipramine (Surmontil)

Indications: Depressive disorders, anxiety disorders.
Preparations: 25, 50, 100 mg capsules.
Dosage:
   Initial dosage: 25 mg qhs, then increase over 1- to 4-week period.
   Average dosage: 150-200 mg/day.
   Dosage Range: 50-300 mg/day.
   Elderly: 25-50 mg qhs (max 200 mg/day).
Therapeutic Levels: Unknown.
Clinical Guidelines: Trimipramine has no significant advantages over other TCAs.

References, see page 115.

Secondary Amine Tricyclic Antidepressants

Desipramine (Norpramin)

Indications: Depressive disorders, anxiety disorders, and chronic pain.
Preparations: 10, 25, 50, 75, 100, 150 mg tablets; 25, 50 mg capsules.
Dosage:
  Initial dosage: 25 mg qhs, then increase over 1- to 4-week period.
  Average dosage: 150-250 mg/day.
  Dosage range: 50-300 mg/day.
  Elderly: 25-100 mg/day (max 200 mg/day).
Half-Life: 12-24 hr.
Therapeutic Levels: 125-300 ng/mL
Clinical Guidelines: Desipramine is one of the least sedating and least anticholinergic TCAs. It should be considered a first-line heterocyclic agents in elderly patients. Some patients may require AM dosing due to mild CNS activation.

Nortriptyline (Pamelor, Aventyl)

Indications: Depressive disorders, anxiety disorders, and chronic pain.
Preparations: 10, 25, 50, 75 mg capsules; 10 mg/5ml liquid concentrate.
Dosage:
  Initial dosage: 25 mg qhs, then increase over 1- to 4-week period.
  Average dosage: 75-150 mg/day.
  Dosage range: 25-150 mg/day.
  Elderly: 10-75 mg/day (max 150 mg/day).
Half-Life: 18-44 hr.
Therapeutic Levels: 50-150 ng/mL
Clinical Guidelines: Nortriptyline is widely used in the treatment of chronic pain. It is one of the least likely TCAs to cause orthostatic hypotension, and it is a good choice for elderly patients who require a TCA. Nortriptyline is the only antidepressant where serum levels appear to be related to response. Patients generally respond at serum levels between 50-150 ng/mL.

Protriptyline (Vivactil)

Indications: Depressive disorders.
Preparations: 5, 10 mg tablets.
Dosage:
  Initial dosage: 5 mg qAM, then increase over several days to weeks.
  Average dosage: 15-40 mg/day.
  Dosage range: 10-60 mg/day.

Elderly: 5 mg tid (max 40 mg/day).
Half-Life: 50-200 hr.
Therapeutic Levels: 75-200 ng/mL
Clinical Guidelines: Protriptyline is the least sedating and most activating TCA. Avoid giving near bedtime because it can cause insomnia. It has no advantage over other TCAs and is not commonly used.

References, see page 115.

Tetracyclic Antidepressants

Amoxapine (Asendin)

Indications: Depressive disorders, especially major depression with psychotic features.
Preparations: 25, 50, 100, 150 mg tablets.
Dosage:
Initial dosage: 25-50 mg qhs, then increase gradually over 1-4 week period.
Average dosage: 200-250 mg/day.
Dosage range: 50-300 mg/day.
Elderly: Start with 25 mg qhs; increase to 50 mg bid-tid (maximum 300 mg/day).
Half-Life: 8 hr.
Therapeutic Levels: 100-250 ng/mL.
Clinical Guidelines:
  A. Amoxapine is related to the antipsychotic loxapine. Blockade of dopamine receptors may produce extrapyramidal symptoms (EPS) due to dopamine antagonism of its metabolite loxapine (eg, dystonia, akathisia, Parkinsonian symptoms). Dopamine receptor blockade can lead to hyperprolactinemia with subsequent gynecomastia, galactorrhea, or amenorrhea.
  B. Amoxapine is associated with higher rates of seizure, arrhythmia, and fatality in overdose than many other antidepressants. The antipsychotic properties of loxapine may be useful in the treatment of major depression with psychotic features. Amoxapine has added risks of dopamine antagonist side effects, such as tardive dyskinesia.

Maprotiline (Ludiomil)

Indications: Depressive disorders.
Preparations: 25, 50, 75 mg tablets.
Dosage:
Initial dosage: 75 mg qhs for 2 weeks, then increase in 25 mg increments over the next few weeks.
Average dosage: 100-150 mg/day .
Dosage range: 50-200 mg/day.
Elderly: Start with 25 mg qhs. Increase to 50-75 qhs (max 100 mg/day).
Half-Life: 21-25 hr.
Therapeutic Levels: 150-300 ng/mL
Clinical Guidelines:
  A. Maprotiline is associated with higher rates of seizure, arrhythmia, and fatality in overdose than many other antidepressants. Avoid medications

that lower seizure threshold, and avoid use in patients with risk of alcohol or sedative/hypnotic withdrawal syndrome. Do not use in patients with a history of seizures.

B. The long half-life may necessitate a longer period of observation after overdose. Maprotiline is rarely used.

References, see page 115.

Monoamine Oxidase Inhibitors

I. Indications
A. Monoamine oxidase inhibitors (MAOIs) are used in the treatment of depressive and anxiety disorders. MAOIs are particularly useful in the treatment of major depression with atypical features, such as mood reactivity, increased appetite, hypersomnia, and sensitivity to interpersonal rejection.

B. These agents also have significant efficacy in anxiety disorders, such as social phobia and panic disorder with agoraphobia and obsessive-compulsive disorder.

C. Given the dietary restrictions and risk of hypertensive crisis, MAOIs are usually used only after conventional treatments have failed.

II. Pharmacology
A. Monoamine oxidase inhibitors irreversibly inhibit the enzyme, monoamine oxidase, located in the central nervous system, gut and platelets, leading to lack of degradation of monoamines.

B. Two weeks are required after discontinuing an MAOI to replenish the body with normal amounts of the monoamine oxidase enzyme.

C. Oral MAOIs inhibit monoamine oxidase in the gut wall (MAO-A), which leads to increased absorption of tyramine. High levels of tyramine can lead to large abrupt increases in blood pressure, known as hypertensive crisis.

III. Clinical Guidelines
A. **Dietary Restrictions:** These agents require patients to adhere to a low tyramine diet in order to avoid a hypertensive crisis.

B. **Dose Titration:** In order to minimize side effects, these agents must be started at a low dose and titrated upward over days to weeks. This is a major disadvantage compared to SSRIs.

C. **Response Time:** These agents require at least 3-4 weeks for an adequate therapeutic trial, and patients may respond after 6-8 weeks.

D. **Efficacy:** May be slightly more effective than other antidepressant treatments, especially with atypical depression.

E. **Clinical Utility:** Given the side-effect profile and dietary restrictions, these agents are generally reserved for use in patients who are refractory to other antidepressant treatments.

IV. Adverse Drug Reactions
A. **Alpha-1 Blockade:** Alpha-1-adrenergic blockade can lead to marked orthostatic hypotension, which is the most common side effect. Orthostatic hypotension can be treated with salt supplements, support hose, or with fludrocortisone. Dizziness and reflex tachycardia may also occur.

B. **Histaminic Blockade:** Antihistaminic properties can lead to sedation and significant weight gain.

C. **Hypertensive Crisis:** Hypertensive crisis from consuming tyramine containing foods is characterized by markedly elevated blood pressure, headache, sweating, nausea and vomiting, photophobia, autonomic instability, chest pain, cardiac arrhythmias, and even coma and death.

D. **Treatment of Hypertensive Crisis:** Treatment involves the use of oral nifedipine while carefully monitoring blood pressure to make sure it does not drop too far. Alternatively, chlorpromazine, 50 mg orally, may be given. If patients present to the emergency room, they can be given phentolamine, 5 mg IV, followed by 0.25-0.5 mg IM every 4 to six hours as indicated.

E. MAOI Diet: Foods to be avoided: Soy sauce, sauerkraut, aged chicken or beef liver, aged cheese, fava beans, air-dried sausage or other meats, pickled or cured meat or fish, overripe fruit, canned figs, raisins, avocados, yogurt, sour cream, meat tenderizer, yeast extracts, caviar, and shrimp paste. Beer and wine are generally contraindicated; however, recent studies indicate that they contain very little tyramine.

F. Pyridoxine Deficiency: Pyridoxine deficiency, manifesting with para-esthesias, may occur and can be treated with vitamin B6, 50 mg per day.

G. Overdose: Overdose can be fatal. Dialysis may be helpful along with supportive treatment. Death may occur from arrhythmias, seizures or renal failure.

H. Surgery: Discontinue MAOIs 14 days before surgery to prevent hypertensive crisis from anesthetics.

I. Mania: MAOIs can induce mania or rapid cycling in patients with bipolar disorder.

J. Comorbid Medical Illness: Use with caution in patients with liver disease, abnormal liver function tests, cardiovascular disease, migraine headaches, renal disease, hyperthyroidism, or Parkinson's disease.

K. Pregnancy: There are very limited data available. It is probably best to avoid use in general. Selegiline is Pregnancy Category C.

L. Miscellaneous: Other side effects include, liver toxicity, agitation, dry mouth, constipation or diarrhea, seizures, sexual dysfunction, insomnia, and edema.

V. Drug Interactions

A. Serotonergic Syndrome: A serotonergic syndrome characterized by nausea, confusion, hyperthermia, autonomic instability, tremor, myoclonus, rigidity, seizures, coma and death, can occur when MAOIs are combined with SSRIs, TCAs, or carbamazepine. Wait fourteen days after discontinuing an MAOI before starting a TCA or SSRI. Discontinue most SSRIs and other antidepressants 14 days before beginning an MAOI. Wait 5-6 weeks after discontinuing fluoxetine because of the long half-life of norfluoxetine. Concurrent use of non-SSRI, non-TCA antidepressants such as bupropion and mirtazapine are contraindicated.

B. Opioids: Opiate analgesics, especially meperidine, may lead to autonomic instability, delirium and death.

C. Sympathomimetics: Sympathomimetic agents such as amphetamines, cocaine, ephedrine, epinephrine, norepinephrine, dopamine, isoproter-enol, St. John's Wort, methylphenidate, oxymetazoline, phenylephrine, and metaraminol can lead to a hypertensive crisis.

D. Antihypertensives: Antihypertensive agents can further increase the likelihood of hypotension.

E. Oral Hypoglycemics: MAOIs can potentiate decreases in blood glucose when combined with oral hypoglycemics.

F. Miscellaneous: MAOIs should be discontinued prior to general anesthesia or local anesthesia containing sympathomimetic vasoconstrictors. Carbamazepine and oxcarbazepine are chemically similar to TCAs and may also trigger a hypertensive crisis. Psychosis has been described with dextromethorphan. Hypertensive reactions have occurred with buspirone.

Phenelzine (Nardil)

Indications: Effective for atypical depression. Also used for anxiety disorders, such as panic disorder with agoraphobia, social phobia, and obsessive-compulsive disorder.
Preparations: 15 mg tablets.
Dosage:
   Initial dosage: 15 mg bid; increase by 15 mg/day each week.
   Average dosage: 30-60 mg/day.
   Dosage range: 15-90 mg/day.
   Elderly: Start with 7.5-15 mg/day; max 60 mg/day.
Therapeutic Levels: Not established.
Clinical Guidelines: Major morbidity and mortality risks are associated with MAOI use. Phenelzine is associated with a higher incidence of weight gain, drowsiness, dry mouth, and sexual dysfunction than tranylcypromine.

Selegiline (ENSAM)

Indications: Major depressive disorder.
Preparations: 6 mg, 9 mg, 12 mg/24hr patches.
Dosage: Initial target dose 6 mg/24hr; may increase in 3 mg/24hr increments after 2 weeks at lower dosage.
   Elderly: 6 mg/24hr.
Therapeutic Levels: Not established.
Clinical Guidelines: Antidepressant activity requires inhibition of MAO-A and MAO-B in the brain. At the 6 mg/24hr dose, the transdermal preparation will not significantly inhibit MAO-A in the GI tract but will inhibit MAO-A and MAO-B in the brain; therefore, at the 6 mg/24hr dose, dietary restrictions are not required. Dietary restrictions are required for 9 mg 12/24hr doses. The most common side effect is skin irritation at the application site.

Tranylcypromine (Parnate)

Indications: Approved for atypical depression. Also used for anxiety disorders, such as panic disorder with agoraphobia, social phobia, and obsessive-compulsive disorder.
Preparations: 10 mg tablets.
Dosage:
   Initial dosage: 10 mg bid. Increase by 10 mg/day each week.
   Average dosage: 20-40 mg/day.
   Dosage range: 10-60 mg/day.
   Elderly: Start with 5-10 mg/day; max 30-40 mg/day.
Therapeutic Levels: Not established.
Clinical Guidelines: Major morbidity and mortality risks are associated with

38 Monoamine Oxidase Inhibitors

MAOI use. Tranylcypromine is associated with less weight gain, drowsiness, dry mouth, and sexual dysfunction than phenelzine. Tranylcypromine is more likely to cause insomnia than phenelzine.

References, see page 115.

Antipsychotics

Clinical Use of Antipsychotics

I. Indications

A. Antipsychotic agents (also referred to as neuroleptics) are indicated for the treatment of schizophrenia and bipolar disorder. Antipsychotics are also used for schizoaffective disorder, mood disorders with psychotic symptoms, and brief psychotic disorder. They often improve functioning in patients with dementia or delirium when psychotic symptoms are present. These agents are also frequently used for treatment of substance-induced psychotic disorders and in psychotic symptoms associated with certain personality disorders (borderline).

II. Pharmacology

A. Typical and atypical antipsychotics are distinguished by the unique receptor-binding profiles of antipsychotics with dopamine and serotonin receptors. While typical antipsychotic agents had been the first-line treatment for schizophrenia, atypical antipsychotics have replaced the typical agents because of their greater tolerability and increased efficacy.

B. The efficacy of typical antipsychotic agents is primarily related to their binding to dopamine D2 receptors.

1. Typical antipsychotic agents may be divided into high-, moderate- and low-potency categories based on their level of dopamine receptor antagonism.

2. All agents within the typical antipsychotic category are equally effective.

   a. High-potency agents have the highest affinity for D2 receptors and are effective at relatively lower doses.

   b. Low-potency agents have lower D2 affinity and require larger doses to elicit an antipsychotic effect.

C. **Atypical agents** (serotonin-dopamine antagonists, SDAs) are distinguished by their prominent antagonism at the serotonin 2A receptor in addition to D2 blockade.

1. The ratio of serotonin to dopamine blockade is generally high for these agents. These agents are also unique in that there appears to be more selectivity for the mesolimbic dopamine pathway, which is thought to be a site of antipsychotic action.

2. There is relatively less action on the nigrostriatal pathway where extrapyramidal side effects are thought to originate.

D. These drugs have a therapeutic dose range that allows for the antipsychotic effect without inducing significant extrapyramidal symptoms.

1. Clozapine is an antagonist of serotonin-2A, alpha-1, dopamine-1, 2, and 4 receptors. Clozapine also possesses significant antihistamine and anticholinergic properties, leading to a side-effect profile similar to that of the typical low-potency agents.

2. Aripiprazole is a unique atypical agent in that it is a partial dopamine agonist (D2 receptor). It is a serotonin 2A receptor antagonist but is also a partial serotonin 1A agonist.

3. Serotonin-dopamine antagonists include risperidone (Risperdal), olan-

zapine (Zyprexa), ziprasidone (Geodon), and quetiapine (Seroquel).

E. Pharmacokinetics

1. After oral absorption, peak plasma levels of antipsychotics usually occur within 2-4 hours. Liquid preparations are absorbed more quickly. IM injections reach peak levels in 30-60 minutes.
2. Antipsychotic agents undergo extensive hepatic metabolism. Typically 50% of the antipsychotic is excreted via the enterohepatic circulation and 50% is excreted through the kidneys.
3. Antipsychotics are 85-90% protein bound and highly lipophilic.
4. Half-lives generally range from 5-50 hours. Steady state plasma levels are established in 4-10 days.
5. **Switching:** When changing to an atypical antipsychotic, switching should employ the cross-titration method. The new medication should be added while the former medication is usually tapered over time (2-3 weeks).

III. Clinical Guidelines

A. Choosing an Antipsychotic Agent

1. In general, the choice of neuroleptic should be made based on past history of neuroleptic response and side effects.
2. Atypical antipsychotics have gained acceptance as first-line drugs for treatment of psychosis. They provide a superior long-term outcome in treatment of schizophrenia compared to typical antipsychotics. At least two weeks of treatment is required before a significant antipsychotic effect is achieved.
3. Patients with tardive dyskinesia (TD) should be considered for treatment with an atypical agent to avoid progression of neurological impairment.
   a. Clozapine is not associated with tardive dyskinesia.
   b. Olanzapine (Zyprexa), risperidone (Risperdal), quetiapine (Seroquel) and ziprasidone (Geodon) have significantly reduced incidences of tardive dyskinesia.

B. Efficacy

1. **Positive Symptoms:** With the exception of clozapine, no differences have been clearly shown in the efficacy of typical and atypical agents in the treatment of positive symptoms (eg, hallucinations, delusions, disorganization). Clozapine is more effective than typical agents.
2. **Negative Symptoms:** Atypical agents may be more effective in the treatment of negative symptoms (eg, affective flattening, anhedonia, avolition) associated with psychotic disorders.
3. **Treatment-Resistant Psychosis:** Clozapine is the only antipsychotic with substantial data to support efficacy in treatment-resistant psychosis. Thirty percent of poor responders to typical agents show significant improvement when treated with clozapine.
4. **Bipolar Disorder:** Quetiapine, olanzapine, aripiprazole, ziprasidone, and risperidone are FDA-approved for the treatment of acute mania. Olanzapine and aripiprazole have an indication for maintenance treatment of bipolar disorder.

IV. Adverse Drug Reactions

A. Side Effects Primarily Associated with Typical Antipsychotics

1. The typical antipsychotics have traditionally been classified according to their potency. Low-potency typical antipsychotic agents and

clozapine have more troublesome side effects than high-potency agents because of greater antagonism of cholinergic, adrenergic and histaminergic receptors.

2. High-potency typical agents, however, have more frequent extra-pyramidal side effects because of potent antagonism of dopamine receptors. The atypical agents generally have much lower antagonism of cholinergic, adrenergic and histaminergic receptors. Side-effect profiles resulting from antagonism of these receptor pathways is summarized as follows:

   a. **Muscarinic (cholinergic):** Dry mouth, constipation, urinary reten-tion, blurred vision, precipitation of narrow angle glaucoma, ECG changes.

   b. **Alpha-1-adrenergic:** Orthostatic hypotension, lightheadedness, tachycardia, sedation and sexual dysfunction.

   c. **Histamine-1:** Sedation, weight gain, fatigue.

   d. **Dopamine-2:** Extrapyramidal Parkinsonian symptoms (eg, dystonic reactions, masked facies, tremor, shuffling gait); hyperprolactinemia (not with clozapine), dystonic reaction, akathisia (restlessness).

   e. **Serotonin-1C:** May mediate weight gain for some atypical agents.

   f. **Non-Specific Side Effects:** Include hyperthermia, hypothermia, hepatitis, jaundice, photosensitivity, lowered seizure threshold, hematologic changes, hepatitis, and rash.

B. **Metabolic Side Effects**

1. Atypical antipsychotics are associated with weight gain type II diabetes and hyperlipidemia. This association has been based primarily on case-series and has led to significant controversy.

2. The FDA has required product labeling for all atypicals to include warnings about the risk of hyperglycemia and diabetes. There have been reports of diabetic ketoacidosis (DKA).

Relative Risk for Metabolic Side Effects			
	Weight gain	**Diabetes**	**Worsening lipid profile**
Clozapine	+++	+	+
Olanzapine	+++	+	+
Quetiapine	++	+/-	+/-
Risperidone	++	+/-	+/-
Ziprasidone	+/-	-	-
Aripiprazole	+/-	-	-

3. Management of the metabolic risk of atypicals starts with routine monitoring. At baseline, weight, waist circumference (at the iliac crest), blood pressure and fasting glucose and lipids should be measured and monitored periodically (see table below).
4. If weight gain, diabetes or hyperlipidemia develop, patients should be switched to atypical agents associated with less risk for metabolic side effects. Lifestyle modifications are always recommended, with a focus on improving dietary habits and fitness. Referral to a wellness program is recommended.

Monitoring Protocol for Patients on Atypical agents (SDAs)*							
	Base-line	4 weeks	8 weeks	12 weeks	Quar-terly	An-nu-ally	Every 5 years
Per-sonal/-family history	X					X	
Weight (BMI)	X	X	X	X	X		
Blood press-ure	X			X			
Fasting plasma glucose	X			X			
Fasting lipid profile	X			X			X

*More frequent assessments may be warranted based on clinical status

C. **Neuroleptic Malignant Syndrome (NMS)** is an uncommon side effect with a possible fatal outcome. NMS is marked by elevated temperature, autonomic instability, delirium, and rigid muscle tone, developing over 24-72 hours. Risk factors for neuroleptic malignant syndrome include dehydration, heat exhaustion, and poor nutrition.
D. **Agranulocytosis** is most common with clozapine (1-2% incidence). Clozapine should be discontinued if the WBC drops below 3,000/mcL or 50% of the patient's normal level, or if the absolute granulocyte count drops below 1,500/mcL.
E. **Tardive Dyskinesia (TD)** is a long-term neurological impairment, primarily limited to patients with a history of chronic typical neuroleptic administration (greater than two months). Tardive dyskinesias may not resolve after discontinuation of the neuroleptic and may be permanent. TD are characterized by involuntary jerking movements of the face, trunk, neck or extremities. Any striated muscle can be affected including the diaphragm. Risk for TD increases by 1% with each year of typical

antipsychotic treatment. Atypical agents have minimal risk for TD. Treatment may include the following:

1. Quantify the degree of neurological dysfunction with the abnormal involuntary movement scale (AIMS).
2. Reduce or stop antipsychotic if possible.
3. If continued antipsychotic is necessary, consider a change to an atypical agent.

F. **Dystonic reactions** are characterized by painful, acute involuntary muscle spasms. They are common side effects of typical antipsychotic agents. Dystonic reactions commonly involve the extremities, neck (torticollis), and ocular muscles (oculogyric crisis). The muscle contractions are not life-threatening unless they involve airway passages (eg, larynx) and lead to airway obstruction. Treatment may include:

1. **Intramuscular or Intravenous Antiparkinsonian Agent**
   a. Benztropine (Cogentin), 1-2 mg PO, IM, IV **OR**
   b. Diphenhydramine (Benadryl), 50 mg PO, IM, IV.
2. Consider change of antipsychotic. Prophylaxis against further episodes of dystonia is accomplished with an oral anticholinergic agent such as benztropine (Cogentin), 2 mg PO bid for 1-2 months. If dystonic reactions occur after discontinuing the anticholinergic agent, longer prophylactic treatment should be provided (eg, 3-6 months).

G. Drug-induced parkinsonian symptoms include bradykinesia, tremor, cogwheel rigidity, masked facies, and shuffling gait. Treatments include:

1. Decreasing antipsychotic dose.
2. Use of anticholinergic drug (eg, benztropine).
3. Changing to lower-potency or atypical agent.
4. Tremor can be treated with propranolol, 10-40 mg PO bid to qid.

H. Akathisia is characterized by an intense sense of restlessness or anxiety. Treatments include:

1. Decreasing antipsychotic dose.
2. Trial of anticholinergic agent (eg, benztropine 2 mg PO bid).
3. Trial of beta-adrenergic antagonist such as propranolol, 10-40 mg PO bid to qid.
4. Consider changing to lower-potency or atypical agent.
5. Trial of benzodiazepine, such as clonazepam, 0.5 mg po bid.

I. **Overdose**

1. Death is uncommon with antipsychotic overdose. Risk of fatality is increased with concurrent use of alcohol or other CNS depressants.
2. Mesoridazine, pimozide and thioridazine are associated with a greatest risk of fatality because of heart block and ventricular tachycardia.
3. CNS depression, hypotension, seizures, fever, ECG changes, hypothermia, and hyperthermia are possible.
4. Treatment may include gastric lavage, catharsis, IV diazepam for treatment of seizure, and medical treatment of hypotension.

J. **Drug Interactions**

1. **Antacids and cimetidine.** Absorption of antipsychotics may be inhibited.
2. **Anticholinergics, antihistamines, antiadrenergics.** Additive effects.
3. **Antihypertensives** may potentiate hypotension; antipsychotics may inhibit neuronal uptake of clonidine.
4. **Anticonvulsants** may induce metabolism and decrease level of

antipsychotic; phenothiazines may decrease metabolism or increase the level of phenytoin.

5. **Antidepressants** (tricyclics and SSRIs) may reduce metabolism and increase levels of antipsychotics.
6. **Antipsychotics** may increase levels of tricyclics.
7. **Barbiturates** may reduce levels of antipsychotics by enzyme induction and may cause respiratory depression.
8. **Bromocriptine** may worsen psychotic symptoms. Antipsychotics will decrease effect of bromocriptine.
9. **Cigarettes** may increase metabolism and decrease level of antipsychotics.
10. **CNS depressants** (including benzodiazepines, narcotics, and alcohol) enhance sedative effects of antipsychotics.
11. **Digoxin** absorption may be increased.
12. **Isoniazid** may increase risk of hepatic toxicity.
13. **L-Dopa.** Effects blocked by dopamine antagonists.
14. **Lithium.** Possible risk of neuroleptic-induced encephalopathic syndrome or neurotoxicity.
15. **MAOIs** will potentiate hypotensive effects of antipsychotics.
16. **Metrizamide** decreases seizure threshold. Avoid concomitant use with typical agents.
17. **Oral Contraceptives** may increase levels of antipsychotics.
18. **Stimulants.** Amphetamine may worsen psychotic symptoms. Antipsychotics will lessen effects of stimulants.
19. **Warfarin.** Highly protein-bound, may alter antipsychotic levels; levels may be decreased, leading to decreased clotting time.

K. **Pre-Existing Medical Conditions**
1. **Cardiac History.** Use high-potency agents (other than pimozide) or atypicals (other than clozapine) to avoid conduction abnormalities. Avoid ziprasidone in patients with QT prolongation.
2. **Elderly** patients are more sensitive to side effects; atypical drugs should be utilized initially. Most experience is with risperidone and quetiapine. If typical agents are used, start with a low dose of a high-potency agent (0.5 mg of haloperidol) and increase slowly.
3. **Hematologic Disorder.** Clozapine is contraindicated.
4. **Hepatic, Renal, Cardiac, Respiratory Disease.** Use antipsychotics with caution; monitor renal, cardiac, and liver function.
5. **Parkinson's Disease.** Atypical agents with lower incidence of EPS (quetiapine, ziprasidone, aripiprazole) are preferred due to selectivity for mesolimbic dopamine tract.
6. **Prostatic Hypertrophy.** Agents with high anticholinergic activity are contraindicated.
7. **Seizure History.** Molindone may have lower seizure risk than other antipsychotics. Atypicals are also indicated for patients with a seizure disorder. Avoid loxapine and clozapine.

8. **Pregnancy.** Typical antipsychotics may slightly increase risk of anomalies. There is insufficient data to evaluate the effect of atypical agents on the fetus. These agents are designated pregnancy category C.

9. **Dementia.** The FDA has found use of atypicals in dementia patients to be associated with increased mortality.

References, see page 115.

Atypical Antipsychotics

I. Indications

A. Atypical antipsychotics are indicated for psychotic disorders, including schizophrenia, schizoaffective disorder, bipolar mania, brief psychotic disorders, and psychotic symptoms associated with mood disorders, substance abuse, organic brain syndromes, dementia, and personality disorders.

B. Olanzapine/Fluoxetine combination and quetiapine are approved for treatment of bipolar depression. Other atypicals are likely to be efficacious for bipolar depression as well. It can also reduce suicide in psychotic patients.

C. Risperidone is indicated for treatment of irritability, aggression, self-injurious behavior, and mood lability in children (ages 5-16) with autism.

D. Clozapine has been demonstrated to be more effective for positive symptoms in treatment-resistant psychotic patients.

II. Pharmacology

A. The primary distinguishing property of the currently available atypical agents (serotonin-dopamine antagonists, SDAs) is prominent antagonism at the serotonin-2A receptor in addition to D2 blockade.

B. The ratio of serotonin to dopamine blockade is generally high for these agents. These agents are unique in that there appears to be more selectivity for the mesolimbic dopamine pathway, which is thought to be important in mediating antipsychotic action.

C. Atypical agents have relatively less action on the nigrostriatal pathway where extrapyramidal side effects are thought to originate. As a group these drugs have a therapeutic dose range that allows for the antipsychotic effect without inducing significant extrapyramidal symptoms.

D. Aripiprazole (Abilify) is a partial dopamine D2 agonist, serotonin 2A antagonist and a serotonin 1A partial antagonist.

E. Clozapine (Clozaril) is an antagonist of serotonin-2A, alpha-1, and dopamine-1, 2, and 4 receptors. Clozapine also possesses significant antihistamine and anticholinergic properties, resulting in a side-effect profile that is similar to that of the typical low-potency agents.

F. Risperidone (Risperdal), olanzapine (Zyprexa), ziprasidone (Geodon) and quetiapine (Seroquel) are other available serotonin-dopamine antagonists.

III. Clinical Guidelines

A. Clozapine should be reserved for patients who have failed to respond to two different antipsychotics.

B. Atypical agents are utilized as first-line treatment for psychosis. Atypical agents are also used if a patient develops significant side effects when treated with typical agents. These agents produce superior long-term outcomes compared to typical agents in the treatment of schizophrenia.

C. Poor response of negative symptoms of psychosis is an indication for a trial of an atypical agent. Some negative symptoms can be caused by treatment with typical neuroleptics. For example, neuroleptic-induced Parkinsonism can be misinterpreted as flat affect. The atypical agents may be efficacious for primary negative symptoms.

D. Patients with tardive dyskinesia (TD) should be considered for treatment with an atypical agent to avoid progression of neurological impairment.

syndrome. Clozapine is often effective against symptoms that are resistant to typical agents. It is more effective than typical agents in treatment of the negative symptoms of schizophrenia.

B. Clozapine can decrease the risk of suicide in schizophrenia and the FDA has approved the indications for clozapine to include suicide prevention. WBC should be monitored weekly for the first 3 months of treatment. Thereafter, monitoring can be reduced to every 2 weeks. If WBC count has been at least 3,500/mcL for one year, the FDA permits monitoring as infrequently as once a month.

III. **Side-Effect Profile:** Orthostatic hypotension (high), sedation (high), anticholinergic (high), extrapyramidal symptoms (absent). Most common side effects are sedation, dizziness, hypotension, tachycardia, constipation, hyperthermia, hypersalivation. Hypersalivation can be treated with anticholinergic agents.

IV. **Contraindications:** Clozapine is contraindicated in patients with granulocytopenia or a history of agranulocytosis induced by clozapine. Do not use clozapine with drugs that suppress bone marrow or have a risk of agranulocytosis (eg, carbamazepine, sulfonamides).

V. **Adverse Effects**

A. Clozapine has a 1-2% incidence of agranulocytosis. Patients should be instructed to promptly report the onset of fever, sore throat, weakness or other signs of infection. Discontinue the drug if the WBC drops below 3,000/mcL, or 50% of patient's normal count, or if granulocyte count drops below 1,500/mcL. Once the WBC normalizes, the patient may be rechallenged. Patient should not be rechallenged if WBC falls below 2,000/mcL or granulocyte count falls below 1,000/mcL.

B. A 5% incidence of seizure has been noted in patients taking more than 600 mg/day of clozapine. If seizures develop, discontinue drug use and consider restarting with concurrent use of divalproex (Depakote).

C. Rare myocarditis (5-100 cases/100,000 patient years) has been seen, especially during, but not limited to the first month of clozapine treatment. Consider myocarditis if patients present with unexplained fatigue, dyspnea, tachypnea, fever, chest pain, palpitations, other signs of heart failure, or ECG changes (ST-T wave abnormalities or arrhythmias).

D. Use clozapine with caution and at low doses in patients with hepatic or renal disease.

E. Monitor patients for hypotension and tachycardia. When discontinuing clozapine, the dosage should be tapered over two weeks because cholinergic rebound may occur.

VI. **Drug Interactions**

A. **Cimetidine (Tagamet)** may increase clozapine levels. Ranitidine (Zantac) should be used instead.

B. **Fluvoxamine** can double clozapine levels due to CYP1A2 inhibition.

C. **TCAs** can increase risk for seizures, cardiac changes, sedation.

Risperidone (Risperdal)

Class: Benzisoxazole.
Mechanism: Antagonist of serotonin-2A, dopamine-2 and alpha-1 receptors.
Preparations: 0.25, 0.5, 1, 2, 3, 4 mg tablets (1 mg tablet is scored); 1 mg/mL oral soln; long-acting IM preparation (Consta): 25, 37.5 mg and 50 mg vials; disintegrating tablet (M-tab): 0.5, 1, and 2 mg tabs.
I. **Dosage**
   A. **Initial Dosage:** 1 mg bid, then increase by 1 mg every 2-3 days to 2-3 mg bid.
   B. **Acute Agitation:** No acute intramuscular dose is available.
   C. **Maintenance:** 2-8 mg bid, many patients can be treated with 4 mg given as a single dose.
   D. **Long-Acting Intramuscular Formulation (Consta):** 25-50 mg IM every month (no evidence to increase beyond 50 mg).
   E. **Elderly:** Reduced dosage (0.5-4 mg/day).
   F. **Metabolism:** Half-life is 3-20 hours. Hepatic metabolism to an active metabolite. Renal clearance. No risperidone-specific drug interactions.
   G. **Therapeutic Level:** Not established.
II. **Clinical Guidelines**
   A. Risperidone is generally very well tolerated. A low incidence of extrapyramidal symptoms is associated with doses less than 6 mg. Risperidone may be given as a once-a-day dose.
   B. There is increasing experience with successful use of risperidone in elderly populations. There have been a number of case reports of neuroleptic malignant syndrome.
III. **Side-Effect Profile**
   A. Orthostatic hypotension and reflex tachycardia (alpha 1 receptor mediated, minimized with slow upward titration), insomnia, and agitation are the most frequent side effects.
   B. The incidence of extrapyramidal symptoms is very low. Risperidone can cause weight gain and increase prolactin levels. Although usually not clinically significant, increased prolactin can be associated with amenorrhea, galactorrhea, gynecomastia, and impotence.

Olanzapine (Zyprexa, Zydis)

Class: Thienobenzodiazepine
Mechanism: Antagonist of serotonin-2A, dopamine-1, 2, 3, 4, alpha-1, histamine-1, and muscarinic-1 receptors.
Preparations: Zyprexa: 2.5, 5, 7.5, 10, 15 mg tablets.
   Zydis: 10, 15 and 20 mg orally disintegrating tablets.
   IM Zyprexa (for acute use) 10 mg. A long-acting formulation is pending FDA approval.
Dosage:
   Initial dosage: 10 mg/day.
   Range: 10-40 mg/day.
   IM: 5 -10 mg IM every 2 hours (maximum dose not determined).
Therapeutic Level: Not established.

I. **Metabolism:** Half-life is 21-50 hours. Hepatic metabolism (primarily through CYP450 1A2) to inactive metabolites. Olanzapine levels are decreased by tobacco use and by carbamazepine (1A2 induction). Olanzapine levels may be increased by fluvoxamine (1A2 inhibition). Dose should be reduced in the elderly. Olanzapine levels tend to be higher in females.

II. **Clinical Guidelines**
   A. Very well tolerated. No titration is required and many patients can be treated with once-a-day dosing. Weight gain can occur. Doses beyond 20 mg/day may be required in many patients because of pharmacokinetic variability.
   B. Patients should be monitored for type II diabetes and hyperlipidemia and other metabolic side effects.

III. **Side-Effect Profile**
   A. Most common side effects are drowsiness, dry mouth, akathisia, and insomnia. Less frequent are orthostatic hypotension, lightheadedness, nausea, and tremor. Weight gain is common with olanzapine as are increases in lipids and plasma glucose.
   B. There are reports of new-onset diabetes and diabetic ketoacidosis. Despite a similar chemical structure to clozapine, there is no evidence of hemotoxicity.

Quetiapine (Seroquel)

Class: Dibenzothiazepine.

Mechanism: Quetiapine (Seroquel) is an antagonist at the serotonin-2A, dopamine-2, alpha-1 and 2, and histamine-1 receptors.

Preparations: 25, 100, 200, and 300 mg tablets.

Dosage:
   Initial dosage for acute psychosis: 100 mg bid, increased by 50-100 mg every 1 to 3 days to a total daily dose of 600-800 mg
   Elderly: Clearance is reduced by 40% in elderly; dosage should be reduced in the elderly.

Therapeutic Level: Not established.

Metabolism: Half-life is 6 hours, hepatic metabolism (CY50 3A4), no active metabolites. Low potential for drug interactions.

I. **Clinical Guidelines**
   A. May be effective for primary negative symptoms of schizophrenia. Well tolerated. No anticholinergic side effects. Very low incidence of extrapyramidal symptoms. No sustained elevation of prolactin. Requires bid or tid dosing. Patients should be monitored for type II diabetes, hyperlipidemia and other metabolic side effects.
   B. There is significant off-label usage of quetiapine at much lower doses for agitation associated with dementia, delirium, anxiety disorders, insomnia and borderline personality disorder. Very little of this practice is evidence based.

II. **Side-Effect Profile**
   A. Orthostatic hypotension may occur during initial dose titration due to alpha-blockade. Somnolence and weight gain may occur. Dyspepsia, abdominal pain, and dry mouth may also occur.

B. There are reports of new onset diabetes and diabetic ketoacidosis.

Ziprasidone (Geodon)

I. **Pharmacology**
   A. **Class:** Benzisothiazolyl piperazine.
   B. **Indications:** Psychotic disorders.
   C. **Mechanism:** D2, D3, 5HT2A, 5HT1A antagonism; also blocks reuptake of monoamines.
   D. **Preparations:** 20, 40, 60 and 80 mg capsules, IM formulation (acute use): 20 mg/mL single-dose vial.
   E. **Maintenance Dosage:** Target dose is 80 mg bid; some patients benefit from doses greater than 160 mg/day.
   F. **IM Preparation:** 10 mg IM every 2 hours or 20 mg IM every 4 hours to maximum daily dose of 40 mg.
   G. **Therapeutic Level:** Not established.
   H. **Metabolism:** Inactive metabolites, half-life 4 hours. Low potential for drug interactions.

II. **Clinical Guidelines**
   A. Very low incidence of extrapyramidal symptoms. Prolactin elevation is minimal. The incidence of weight gain, lipid abnormalities and glucose intolerance is lower than that seen with other atypical antipsychotics.
   B. While there are no reports linking ziprasidone to cardiac arrhythmias, caution should be exercised in patients with pre-existing increased QT interval (from medications or cardiac disease). These patients should have a baseline ECG. QT prolongation has not been observed with the IM formulation.
   C. **Side-Effect Profile:** Dizziness, nausea, and postural hypotension are the most common side effects. Prolactin elevation can occur. Sedation is more common with the IM preparation.

References, see page 115.

High-Potency Antipsychotics

Side-Effect Profile: Orthostatic hypotension, sedation, and anticholinergic. Extrapyramidal symptoms are frequent.
Clinical Guidelines: High-potency agents have less sedative, hypotensive and anticholinergic side effects. Many patients require concurrent use of an antiparkinsonian agent (eg, benztropine) to control extrapyramidal symptoms. Due to diminishing use of these medications, availability of dosage forms and strengths may be limited.

Fluphenazine (Prolixin)

Class: Piperazine.
Indications: Psychotic disorders.
Preparations: 1, 2.5, 5, 10 mg tablets; 2.5, 5 mg/mL oral solution; 2.5 mg/mL parenteral solution (IM); 25 mg/mL decanoate (IM).
Dosage:
    Initial: 2.5-10 mg/day, may be titrated to 40 mg/day.
    Maintenance: 10-20 mg/day.
    Acute agitation: 2.5-5 mg IM, should not exceed daily dose of 10 mg IM
    Elderly: 0.5-2mg bid/tid.
    Chronic noncompliance: Switch to decanoate formulation. Give 12.5 mg IM of decanoate every two weeks for every 10 mg of oral dose.
Potency: (equivalent to 100 mg chlorpromazine): 2 mg.
Metabolism: Hepatic metabolism, half-life 10-20 hours. The decanoate formulation has a typical duration of action of 2 weeks.
Therapeutic Level: Not established.
Clinical Guidelines: Decanoate formulation available. Use of anticholinergic medication for EPS is common.

Haloperidol (Haldol)

Class: Butyrophenone
Indications: Psychotic disorders, Tourette's Syndrome.
Preparations:
Haloperidol tablets: 0.5, 1, 2, 5, 10, 20 mg.
Haloperidol lactate: 2 mg/mL conc. (PO), 5 mg/mL soln. (IM- for acute use).
Haloperidol decanoate: 50, 100 mg/mL (IM - depot).
Dosage:
    Initial: 5-10 mg/day.
    Maintenance: 5-20 mg/day.
    Acute agitation: 5.0 - 10 mg IM. Should not exceed daily dose of 20 mg IM.
    Elderly: 0.5-2 mg bid/tid.
    Chronic noncompliance: Switch to haloperidol decanoate at 10-20 times

the daily dose, given on monthly basis. Maximum initial dose of 100 mg/day IM. Give balance of dose 4-5 days later if necessary. Do not give more than 3 mL per injection site.

Tourette's disorder in children: 0.05- 0.1 mg/kg in 2 or 3 divided doses
Potency: (equivalent to 100 mg chlorpromazine): 2 mg
Metabolism: Hepatic metabolism to active metabolite. Half-life 10–20 hours. Duration of action of decanoate is approximately 4 weeks.
Therapeutic Level: 5-20 ng/mL.
Clinical Guidelines: High incidence of extrapyramidal symptoms.

Pimozide (Orap)

Class: Diphenylbutylpiperidine.
Indications: Psychotic disorders, Tourette's Syndrome.
Preparations: 2.0 mg tablets.
Dosage:
   Tourette's: 0.5-1 mg bid, then increase dose every other day as needed (max 0.2 mg/kg/day or 10 mg).
   Antipsychotic maintenance: 1-10 mg/day.
Potency (equivalent to 100 mg chlorpromazine): 1 mg.
Metabolism: Hepatic metabolism. Half-life 55 hours.
Therapeutic Level: Not established.
Contraindications: Pimozide is contraindicated in patients with a history of cardiac arrhythmia or with drugs that prolong QT interval.
Major Safety Concerns: Clinical Guidelines: Pimozide may cause ECG changes, including prolongation of QT interval, T-wave inversion, and appearance of U waves and alter effects of antiarrhythmic agents. Cardiac side effects of pimozide make haloperidol safer first-line treatment for Tourette's Syndrome. Use caution in patients with a history of hypokalemia. Not commonly used for psychosis.

Thiothixene (Navane)

Class: Thioxanthene.
Indications: Psychotic disorders.
Preparations: Capsules: 1, 2, 5, 10, 20 mg.
Thiothixene hydrochloride: 5 mg/mL oral solution; 5 mg/mL parenteral (IM).
Dosage:
   Initial dosage: 2-5 mg bid-tid. Titrate to 20-40 mg/day (max 60 mg/day).
   Maintenance: 5-20 mg/day.
   Acute agitation: 5 mg IM 4 hour prn.
   Elderly: 1-15 mg/day.
Potency (equivalent to 100 mg chlorpromazine): 5 mg.
Metabolism: Hepatic metabolism. Half-life 10-20 hours.
Therapeutic Level: Not established. Some suggest 2-57 ng/mL.
Clinical Guidelines: May produce ocular pigmentary changes. Periodic ophthalmological examination is recommended. Akathisia is commonly seen with this medication, which can be refractory to anticholinergic treatment.

Trifluoperazine (Stelazine)

Class: Piperazine.
Preparations: 1, 2, 5, 10 mg tablets; 10 mg/mL oral solution, 2 mg/mL soln. (IM).
Dosage:
   Initial: 2-5 mg bid-tid. Titrate to 20-40 mg/day (max 60 mg/day).
   Maintenance: 5-20 mg/day.
   Acute agitation: 5 mg IM q 4 hour prn (max of 20 mg/day). Do not repeat dosage in less than 4 hrs.
   Elderly: 1-15 mg/day.
Potency (equivalent to 100 mg chlorpromazine): 5 mg.
Metabolism: Hepatic metabolism. Half-life 10–20 hours.
Therapeutic Level: Not established.
Clinical Guidelines: Associated with few ECG changes.

References, see page 115.

Mid-Potency Antipsychotics

Side-Effect Profile: Orthostatic hypotension (moderate), sedation (moderate), anticholinergic (moderate), extrapyramidal symptoms (high). Anticholinergic side effects of mid-potency agents lessen the need for medication to control extrapyramidal side effects. Neuroleptic malignant syndrome, tardive dyskinesia, and dystonic reactions are possible. Due to diminishing use of these medications, availability of dosage forms and strengths may be limited.

Loxapine (Loxitane)

Class: Dibenzoxapine.
Preparations: 5, 10, 25, 50 mg capsules; 25 mg/mL oral solution: 50 mg/mL parenteral solution (IM).
Dosage:
　　Initial dosage: 10 mg bid. Titrate as needed to max of 250 mg/day in divided doses.
　　Maintenance: 50-100 mg/day.
　　Acute agitation: 12.5-50 mg IM q4-6h prn.
　　Elderly: 5-25 mg/day.
Potency (equivalent to 100 mg chlorpromazine): 12.5 mg.
Metabolism: Hepatic metabolism to active metabolite. Half-life 5-15 hours.
Therapeutic Level: Not established.
Clinical Guidelines: Loxapine may be associated with a higher risk of seizure than other high- and mid-potency agents. Concurrent use with medications that lower the seizure threshold should be avoided or in patients at risk for seizures.

Molindone (Moban)

Class: Dihydroindole
Preparations: 5, 10, 25, 100 mg tablets; 20 mg/mL conc. (PO).
Dosage:
　　Initial: 15-20 mg tid. Titrate to 10-40 mg tid-qid (max 225 mg/day).
　　Maintenance: 50-100 mg/day.
Potency (equivalent to 100 mg chlorpromazine): 10 mg.
Metabolism: Hepatic metabolism, half-life 10–20 hours.
Therapeutic Level: Not established.
Clinical Guidelines: Studies suggest molindone is associated with less weight gain, amenorrhea, and impotence than other typical antipsychotics. Molindone appears less likely to cause seizures than other antipsychotics.

Perphenazine (Trilafon)

Class: Piperazine.
Preparations: 2, 4, 8, 16 mg tablets; 16 mg/5 mL oral solution; 5 mg/mL parenteral solution (IM).
Dosage:
   Initial: 4-8 mg tid, titrate to 8-16 mg bid-tid (max 64 mg/day).
   Maintenance: 4-40 mg/day.
   Acute agitation: 5-10 mg IM q 6h. prn (max 30 mg/day).
Potency (equivalent to 100 mg chlorpromazine): 10 mg.
Metabolism: Hepatic metabolism, half-life 10-20 hours.
Therapeutic Level: Not established.
Clinical Guidelines: Perphenazine has antiemetic properties.

References, see page 115.

Low-Potency Antipsychotics

Side-Effect Profile: High potentiation of anticholinergic, antihistaminic, anti-adrenergic agents. Orthostatic hypotension (moderate), sedation (high), anticholinergic (moderate), extrapyramidal symptoms (low). Neuroleptic malignant syndrome, tardive dyskinesia, and dystonic reactions are possible. Higher risk than most other antipsychotics for ECG changes (including T-wave changes), jaundice, decreased libido, and retrograde ejaculation. Due to diminishing use of these medications, availability of dosage forms and strengths may be limited.

Chlorpromazine (Thorazine)

Class: Aliphatic Phenothiazine.
Preparations:
Tablets: 10, 25, 50, 100, 200 mg; Slow-release capsules: 30, 75, 100, 200, 300 mg. Oral liquid preparations: 30 mg/mL and 100 mg/mL conc; 10 mg/5 mL syrup. Parenteral injection: 25 mg/mL (IM). Suppositories: 25, 100 mg (PR).
Dosage:
    Initial: 10-50 mg PO bid-qid, titrate to 200-800 mg/day in divided doses (max 2000 mg/day).
    Acute agitation: 25-50 mg IM q 4-6h.
    Maintenance: 200-800 mg/day.
    Elderly: Not recommended due to orthostatic hypotension.
Potency (equivalent to 100 mg chlorpromazine): 100 mg.
Metabolism: Hepatic metabolism to many metabolites.
Therapeutic Level: Not useful due to many active metabolites.
    A. Major Safety Concerns
    Higher risk than most other typical antipsychotics for seizure, cholestatic jaundice, photosensitivity, skin discoloration (bluish), and granular deposits in lens and cornea. Prolongation of QT and PR intervals, blunting of T-waves, ST segment depression can occur. Associated with a high incidence of hypotensive and anticholinergic side effects.
    B. Chlorpromazine has high lethality in overdose. It has a higher risk than many other antipsychotics for life-threatening agranulocytosis. Use chlorpromazine with caution in patients with a history of cardiovascular, liver, or renal disease. Avoid use in pregnancy (especially in first trimester).
Clinical Guidelines:
Can be used for treatment of nausea or vomiting (10-25 mg po qid; 25 mg IM qid; 100 mg suppository tid) and intractable hiccups (25-50 mg qid).

Mesoridazine (Serentil)

Class: Piperidine
Preparations: 10, 25, 50, 100 mg tablets; 25 mg/mL oral solution; 25 mg/mL parenteral solution (IM).
Dosage:
    Initial: 25-50 mg po tid. Titrate to 300 mg/day (max 400 mg/day).
    Acute agitation: 25-50 mg IM. Dose may be repeated q 4-6 hour.
    Maintenance: 100-400 mg/day.
    Elderly: Avoid because of hypotension risk.
Potency (equivalent to 100 mg chlorpromazine): 50 mg.
Metabolism: Hepatic metabolism to many metabolites. Half-life 24-48 hours.
Therapeutic Level: Not established.
Major Safety Concerns: Because of its association with QT prolongation and subsequent increased risk for fatal arrhythmias, mesoridazine is reserved for only those patients who have not responded to other antipsychotic agents.

Thioridazine (Mellaril)

Class: Piperidine
Preparations: 10, 15, 25, 50, 100, 150, 200 mg tablets; 5 mg/mL, 30 mg/mL and 100 mg/mL oral solution.
Dosage:
    Initial dosage: 25-100 mg tid; titrate to 100-400 mg bid (max 800 mg/day)
    Maintenance: 200-800 mg/day; never exceed 800 mg/day. No IM form available.
    Elderly: avoid because of hypotension risk.
Potency (equivalent to 100 mg chlorpromazine): 100 mg.
Metabolism: Hepatic metabolism to active metabolites including mesoridazine, half-life 10-20 hours.
Therapeutic Level: Not established.
Major Safety Concerns: Because of the association of thioridazine with significant QT prolongation and subsequent increased risk for fatal arrhythmias, thioridazine is reserved for only those patients who have not responded to other antipsychotic agents. Permanent pigmentation of the retina (retinitis pigmentosa) and potential blindness occurs with doses above 800 mg/day. Life-threatening agranulocytosis rarely occurs. Retrograde ejaculation occurs more frequently with thioridazine.

References, see page 115.

Anxiolytics

Anxiolytic medications are used for the treatment of anxiety. Some have shown efficacy in the treatment of specific anxiety disorders. Antidepressants are also used in the treatment of anxiety disorders.

Benzodiazepines

I. Indications
  A. Benzodiazepines are used for the treatment of specific anxiety disorders, such as Panic Disorder, Social Phobia, Generalized Anxiety Disorder, and Adjustment Disorder with Anxious Mood (anxiety due to a specific stressful life event). All anxiolytic benzodiazepines can cause sedation.

II. Pharmacology
  A. Benzodiazepines bind to benzodiazepine receptor sites, which are part of the GABA receptor. Benzodiazepine binding facilitates the action of GABA at the GABA receptor complex, which surrounds a chloride ion channel. GABA binding causes chloride influx into the neuron, with subsequent neuroinhibition.

  B. The benzodiazepines differ in their absorption rates, lipid solubility, metabolism and half-lives. These factors affect the onset of action, duration of action, drug interactions and side-effect profile.

  C. The long half-life of diazepam, chlordiazepoxide, clorazepate, halazepam and prazepam (>100 hrs) is due to the active metabolite desmethyldiazepam.

  D. Most benzodiazepines are metabolized via the microsomal cytochrome P450 system in the liver. Hepatic metabolism involves discreet families of isozymes within the cytochrome system, and most benzodiazepines are metabolized by the 3A4 isoenzyme family. Notable exceptions to this are lorazepam, oxazepam, and temazepam.

III. Clinical Guidelines
  A. Non-psychiatric causes of anxiety, including medical disorders, medications and substances of abuse, should be excluded before beginning benzodiazepine treatment.

  B. Selection of a benzodiazepine should be based on the patient's past response to medication, family history of medication response, medical conditions, current medications (drug interactions), and whether a long half-life or short half-life drug is required. Long half-life drugs can be given less frequently, and they have less serum fluctuation and less severe withdrawal. These agents have a higher potential for drug accumulation and daytime sedation.

  C. The initial dosage should be low and titrated up as necessary, especially when using long half-life drugs, since these may accumulate with multiple dosing over several days. The therapeutic dose for benzodiazepines is far below the lethal dose. Long-term use of benzodiazepines is associated with tolerance and dependence. Continued use of benzodiazepines for more than 3 weeks is associated with tolerance, dependence and a withdrawal syndrome.

1. Tolerance develops most readily to the sedative side effect of benzodiazepines.
2. Cross-tolerance may develop between benzodiazepines and other sedative hypnotic drugs, including alcohol.
3. Withdrawal symptoms include heightened anxiety, tremor, tremors, muscle twitching, sweating, insomnia, tachycardia, hypertension with postural hypotension, and seizures.

D. Avoidance of an abstinence syndrome requires gradual tapering upon discontinuation. One-fourth of the dose per week is a general guideline.

IV. Adverse Drug Reactions

A. **Side Effects:** The most common side effect is sedation. Dizziness, ataxia and impaired fine motor coordination can also occur. Some patients complain of cognitive impairment. Anterograde amnesia has been reported, especially with benzodiazepines that reach peak levels quickly.

B. **Respiratory depression** is rarely an issue, even in patients who overdose on benzodiazepines alone. However, patients who overdose with benzodiazepines and other sedative-hypnotics (commonly alcohol) may experience respiratory depression. Patients with compromised pulmonary function are more sensitive to this effect and even therapeutic doses may cause respiratory impairment.

C. Diazepam (Valium) and chlordiazepoxide (Librium) should not be used in patients with hepatic dysfunction because their metabolism will be impaired and toxicity risk increases.

D. Clonazepam should be avoided in patients with renal dysfunction because the metabolism of clonazepam will be impaired and the risk of toxicity will be high.

V. Drug Interactions

A. The concomitant use of benzodiazepines and other CNS depressant agents, including sedative-hypnotics, will enhance sedation and increase the risk of respiratory depression. Alcohol use should be limited.

B. Most benzodiazepines are metabolized via the liver enzyme CYP3A4; therefore, any other drug also metabolized via this pathway may increase the level of the benzodiazepine (except lorazepam, oxazepam, and temazepam). Other agents that increase benzodiazepine levels include cimetidine, fluoxetine, ketoconazole, metoprolol, propranolol, estrogens, alcohol, erythromycin, disulfiram, valproic acid, nefazodone, and isoniazid. Benzodiazepine levels may be decreased by carbamazepine, rifampin (enzyme induction), and antacids (absorption).

References, see page 115.

Alprazolam (Xanax, Xanax XR, Niravam)

Indications: Panic Disorder, Social Phobia. Can be used in Generalized Anxiety Disorder (GAD) and Adjustment Disorder with Anxious Mood.
Preparations: 0.25, 0.5, 1, 2 mg scored tablets: extended release (XR): 0.5, 1, 2, 3 mg tablets; orally disintegrating: 0.25, 0.5, 1, 2 mg tablets.
Dosage: 0.25-2 mg tid-qid. XR formulation allows for once-daily dosing.
   Elderly: Reduce dosage.
Half-Life: Up to 12 hours. The clinical duration of action is short despite moderate serum half-life.
Clinical Guidelines
  A. Fast onset provides quick relief of acute anxiety. Alprazolam has a relatively short duration of action and multiple dosing throughout the day is required (some patients require as much as qid dosing). It is associated with less sedation but a high incidence of inter-dose anxiety.
  B. The XR formulation is not associated with inter-dose anxiety but will not prevent the development of withdrawal symptoms upon abrupt discontinuation (because half-life is unchanged). Dependence and withdrawal are serious problems with this drug. Since SSRIs and other antidepressants are as effective in anxiety disorders, alprazolam is no longer a first-line drug for the treatment of anxiety disorders.
Pregnancy: Category D.

Chlordiazepoxide (Librium, Libritabs)

Indications: Anxiety and alcohol withdrawal.
Preparations: 5, 10, 25 mg capsules.
Dosage:
   Anxiety: 5-25 mg tid-qid.
   Alcohol withdrawal: 25-50 mg every 2-4 hours (maximum 400 mg/day) prn.
   Dose range: 10-100 mg/day.
   Elderly: Avoid use.
Half-Life: >100 hrs.
Clinical Guidelines: This drug will accumulate with multiple dosing. Because this drug is metabolized by P450 isoenzymes, metabolism can be slowed in the elderly and patients with hepatic impairment. If used for anxiety, once-a-day dosing may be possible. Slower onset of action than Valium.

Clonazepam (Klonopin)

Indications: Approved as an anticonvulsant. Used in Panic Disorder, Social Phobia and general anxiety. Useful in acute treatment of Mania.
Preparations: 0.5, 1, 2 mg tablets; disintegrating wafer: 0.125, 0.25, 0.5, 1, 2 mg wafers.
Dosage:
   Anxiety: 0.25-6 mg q day, in divided dose bid-tid.
   Mania: 0.25-10 mg q day, in divided dose bid-tid.

Elderly: 0.25-1.5 mg q day.
Half-Life: 20-50 hrs. No active metabolites.
Clinical Guidelines: Rapid onset provides prompt relief. Clonazepam, has a long half-life and may be substituted for shorter acting benzodiazepines, such as alprazolam, in the treatment of benzodiazepine withdrawal and panic disorder. The long half-life of clonazepam allows for once-a-day dosing.
Pregnancy: Category D.

Clorazepate (Tranxene)

Indications: Anxiety.
Preparations: 3.75, 7.5, 15 mg tablets; SD (extended release): 11.25, 22.5 mg tablets.
Pharmacology: Clorazepate is metabolized to desmethyldiazepam in the GI tract and absorbed in this active form.
Dosage:
  Anxiety: 7.5 mg tid or 15 mg qhs. Increase as needed; extended-release form can be used once daily.
  Dose range: 15-60 mg/day (maximum 90 mg/day).
  Elderly: Avoid use in the elderly.
Half-Life: >100 hrs.
Clinical Guidelines: This drug will accumulate with multiple dosing and over time. Because this drug is metabolized by P450 isoenzymes, metabolism can be slowed in the elderly and patients with hepatic impairment. If used for anxiety, once-a-day dosing may be possible.

Diazepam (Valium)

Indications: Anxiety, alcohol withdrawal.
Preparations: 2, 5, 10 mg tablets; 15 mg capsules (sustained release); 5 mg/mL solution for IV use. IM administration is not recommended due to erratic incomplete absorption.
Dosage:
  Anxiety: 2-40 mg/day divided bid-tid.
  Alcohol withdrawal: 5-10 mg q 2-4 hr prn withdrawal signs for first 24 hrs, then slow taper. Maximum of 60 mg/day.
  Dose range: 2-60 mg/day.
  Elderly: Use with caution because metabolism is significantly delayed.
Half-Life: 100 hrs.
Clinical Guidelines: Due to its long half-life, it will accumulate with multiple dosing. Because this drug is metabolized by CYP 450 isoenzymes, metabolism can be slowed in the elderly and patients with hepatic impairment. If used for anxiety, once-a-day dosing may be possible.

Lorazepam (Ativan)

Indications: Anxiety, alcohol withdrawal, and adjunct in the treatment of acute psychotic agitation.
Preparations: 0.5, 1, 2 mg tablets; 2 mg/mL, 4 mg/mL soln (IV, IM).
Lorazepam is the only benzodiazepine available in IM form that has rapid, complete, predictable absorption.
Dosage:
  Anxiety: 0.5-6 mg/day (divided doses).
  Alcohol withdrawal: 0.5-2 mg q 2-4 hr prn signs of alcohol withdrawal; or 0.5-1.0 mg IM to initiate treatment. Maximum dose of 10 mg/day.
  Elderly: Metabolism is not significantly affected by age; elderly may be more susceptible to side effects.
Half-Life: 15 hrs. No active metabolites.
Clinical Guidelines:
  A. Metabolism is not P450 dependent and will only be affected when hepatic dysfunction is severe. The inactive glucuronide is renally excreted; it is the benzodiazepine of choice in patients with serious or multiple medical conditions. The metabolism of lorazepam is not affected by age. These properties make it ideal for alcohol withdrawal in a patient with liver dysfunction or who is elderly.
  B. Since the half-life is relatively short, accumulation with multiple dosing usually does not occur. The IM form is useful in rapid control of agitation, resulting from psychosis, or drug-induced agitation. It is also widely used on an oral basis as a prn adjunct to fixed doses of antipsychotic medication.
Pregnancy: Category D.

References, see page 115.

Non-Benzodiazepine Anxiolytics

Buspirone (BuSpar)

Category: Anxiolytic. Non-benzodiazepine, non-sedative hypnotic.
Mechanism: Serotonin 1A agonist.
Indications: Generalized Anxiety Disorder (GAD). May be used to augment antidepressant treatment of Major Depressive Disorder and Obsessive-Compulsive Disorder (OCD). Often useful in the treatment of aggression and agitation in dementia and in patients with developmental disabilities.
Preparations: 5, 10, 15 and 30 mg tablets (15 mg and 30 mg tablets are scored for bisection or trisection).
Dosage:
   Initial Dosage: 7.5 mg bid, then increase by 5 mg every 2-3 days as tolerated.
   Dose Range: 30-60 mg/day (maximum 60 mg/day).
   Elderly: 15-60 mg/day.
   Antidepressant Augmentation: 15-60 mg/day if a patient has a suboptimal response to a 4-6 week trial of an antidepressant.
Half-Life: 2-11 hours. No active metabolites.
Side Effects: Dizziness, headache, GI distress, fatigue.
Clinical Guidelines:
   A. Buspirone lacks the sedation and dependence associated with benzodiazepines, and it causes less cognitive impairment than the benzodiazepines. It is less effective in patients who have taken benzodiazepines in the past because it lacks the euphoria and sedation that these patients may expect.
   B. Unlike benzodiazepines, buspirone does not immediately relieve anxiety. Onset of action may take 2 weeks. The patient may be started on a benzodiazepine and buspirone for two weeks, followed by slow tapering of the benzodiazepine.
Pregnancy: Category B.

Hydroxyzine (Atarax, Vistaril)

Category: Antihistamine, mild anxiolytic.
Mechanism: Histamine receptor antagonist, mild anticholinergic activity.
Indications: Anxiety (short-term treatment), sometimes used to augment the sedative side effects of antipsychotics when given for acute agitation.
Preparations: 10, 25, 50, 100 mg tablets; 10 mg/5 mL syrup; 50 mg/mL solution (IM, not IV).
Dosage:
   Anxiety: 50-100 PO q 4-6 hrs.
   Acute agitation: 50-100 mg IM q 4-6 hrs.
Side Effects: Dry mouth, dizziness, drowsiness, tremor, thickening of bronchial secretions, hypotension, decreased motor coordination.

Drug Interactions: The sedative effect of hydroxyzine will be enhanced by the concomitant use of other sedative drugs. Similarly, the mild anticholinergic properties may be enhanced if another medication with anticholinergic properties is also taken.

Clinical Guidelines: Hydroxyzine is not associated with dependence. It is a weak anxiolytic and only effective for short-term treatment of anxiety. It can be helpful as an adjunct to antipsychotic medications since it will potentiate the sedative side effects and reduce the risk of extrapyramidal side effects.

References, see page 115.

Benzodiazepine Hypnotics 67

Benzodiazepine Hypnotics

Hypnotic medications are used for the treatment of insomnia. Choice of agent is determined by half-life. Short-acting hypnotics are best for the treatment of initial insomnia or difficulties with sleep onset. They are associated with less morning sedation. Long-acting agents are more useful for the treatment of late insomnia or difficulties in maintaining sleep. Long-acting agents are more likely to be associated with daytime sedation. Non-benzodiazepine hypnotics are now widely used and are becoming the treatment of choice versus the benzodiazepine hypnotics

I. **Indications**. Insomnia.
II. **Pharmacology**
   A. The major difference between the anxiolytic and hypnotic benzodiazepines is the rate of absorption.
   B. Benzodiazepine hypnotics are rapidly absorbed from the GI tract and achieve peak serum levels quickly, resulting in rapid onset of sedation.
III. **Clinical Guidelines**
   A. Hypnotics are recommended for short-term use only. Insomnia treatment should include exercise, stress reduction, sleep hygiene, and caffeine avoidance.
   B. Prolonged use of benzodiazepines (generally greater than 3 weeks) is associated with tolerance, dependence and withdrawal syndromes.
   C. The choice of benzodiazepine hypnotic is usually dictated by the need for sleep onset or sleep maintenance, half-life, and drug interactions.
IV. **Adverse Drug Reactions**
   A. Daytime sedation or morning "hangover" is a major complaint when patients take hypnotics with long half-lives. Dizziness and ataxia may occur during the daytime or if the patient awakens during the night. Anterograde amnesia has also been reported.
   B. Benzodiazepines may depress respiration at high doses. Patients with compromised pulmonary function are more sensitive to this effect.
V. **Drug Interactions**
   A. Other CNS depressant agents, including alcohol and sedative-hypnotics will enhance the sedative effect of hypnotic benzodiazepines.
   B. Since triazolam, estazolam, flurazepam, diazepam and quazepam are metabolized via the liver enzyme, CYP3A4, concomitant use of medications that inhibit 3A4 will increase the half-life and potential for toxicity. Inhibitors of CYP3A4 include erythromycin, nefazodone, and ketoconazole.

Estazolam (ProSom)

Indications: Insomnia.
Preparations: 1, 2 mg tablets.
Dosage:
   Insomnia: 1-2 mg qhs

Elderly: 0.5-1.0 mg qhs.
Half-Life: 17 hrs.
Clinical Guidelines: Fast onset of action is useful for treatment of early insomnia. Medium half-life should help patients stay asleep throughout the night. Estazolam offers no real advantage over temazepam (Restoril). Estazolam is not commonly used.

Flurazepam (Dalmane)

Indications: Insomnia.
Preparations: 15, 30 mg capsules.
Dosage: Insomnia: 15-30 mg qhs, less in elderly.
Half-Life: 100 hrs.
Clinical Guidelines: Fast onset is useful in the treatment of early insomnia. Long duration is useful in the treatment of late insomnia, but may result in morning sedation. Shorter half-life medications are preferable to flurazepam, especially in the elderly.

Quazepam (Doral)

Indications: Insomnia.
Preparations: 7.5, 15 mg tablets.
Dosage:
    Insomnia: 7.5-30 mg qhs.
    Elderly: 7.5 mg qhs.
Half-Life: 100 hrs.
Clinical Guidelines: Long duration of action may result in morning sedation. It has no unique properties and is not commonly used.

Temazepam (Restoril)

Indication: Insomnia.
Preparations: 7.5, 15, 30 mg capsules.
Dosage: Insomnia: 7.5-30 mg qhs (less for elderly).
Half-Life: 10-12 hrs.
Clinical Guidelines: Short duration of action limits morning sedation.

Triazolam (Halcion)

Indication: Insomnia.
Preparations: 0.125, 0.25 mg tablets.
Dosage: Insomnia: 0.125-0.25 mg qhs. Reduce dosage in elderly.
Half-Life: 2-3 hrs.

Clinical Guidelines: Ultra-short half-life results in minimal AM sedation. It is best for sleep initiation. Patients may report waking up after 3-4 hours when blood level drops. Triazolam is not recommended for patients who have trouble maintaining sleep throughout the night. Use should be limited to 10 days. Use with caution in the elderly.

References, see page 115.

Non-Benzodiazepine Hypnotics

Chloral Hydrate (Noctec, Somnote)

Category: Sedative-hypnotic.
Mechanism: CNS depression, specific mechanism is unknown.
Indications: Insomnia.
Preparations: 500 mg capsules.
Dosage: 500-1000 mg qhs (short-term only).
Half-Life: 8 hrs.
Clinical Guidelines: Tolerance and dependence regularly develop with consistent use. It is highly lethal in overdose and can cause hepatic and renal damage. The use of chloral hydrate has decreased because benzodiazepines are equally effective and are much safer.
Side Effects: Nausea, vomiting, diarrhea, daytime sedation and impaired coordination.
Interactions: IV furosemide may cause flushing and labile blood pressure. Additive effects when given with other CNS depressants.

Diphenhydramine (Benadryl)

Category: Antihistamine.
Mechanism: Histamine receptor antagonist (sedation), acetylcholine receptor antagonist (extrapyramidal symptom control).
Indications: Mild insomnia, neuroleptic-induced extrapyramidal symptoms, antihistamine.
Preparations: 25, 50 mg tablets; 25, 50 mg capsules; 10 mg/mL and 50 mg/mL soln. (IM, IV), 12.5 mg/5 mL elixir (PO).
Dosage:
  Insomnia: 50 mg PO qhs.
  Extrapyramidal symptoms: 25-50 mg PO bid, for acute extrapyramidal. symptoms 25-50 mg IM or IV.
Half-Life: 1-4 hrs.
Clinical Guidelines: Diphenhydramine is a very weak sedative, and it is minimally effective as a hypnotic. It is non-addicting.
Side Effects: Dry mouth, dizziness, drowsiness, tremor, thickening of bronchial secretions, hypotension, decreased motor coordination, GI distress. May cause exacerbation of narrow angle glaucoma and prostatic hypertrophy.
Drug Interactions: Diphenhydramine has an additive effect when used with other sedatives and other medications with anticholinergic activity. MAOI use is contraindicated within 2 weeks of diphenhydramine.

Eszopiclone (Lunesta)

Category: Non-benzodiazepine hypnotic.
Mechanism: Binds to the GABA receptor but is a non-benzodiazepine.
Indications: Insomnia.
Preparations: 1,2, 3 mg tablets.
Dosage: 2-3 mg qhs (1-2 mg for elderly).
Half-Life: 6 hours.
Clinical Guidelines:
   Eszopiclone has a rapid onset of action. It is especially useful for initiating
   sleep but has a longer duration of action compared to zolpidem CR
   (Ambien CR) and zaleplon (Sonata).
   Eszopiclone is not associated with dependance or withdrawal. The efficacy
   of eszopiclone has been demonstrated in studies lasting 6 months.
Side Effects: Unpleasant taste, headaches, dizziness.
Drug Interactions: Potentiation of other CNS depressants (eg, alcohol). Higher
serum levels have been reported in patients with severe hepatic impairment,
and the dose should be reduced to 1 mg in these individuals. No dose
adjustment is required in patients with mild-to-moderate hepatic impairment or
any degree of renal impairment. Drugs that inhibit CYP3A4 such as
ketoconzaole can elevate eszopiclone plasma levels. Drugs that inhibit CYP3A4
such as rifampin can decrease eszopiclone plasma levels. Drugs that induce
CYP3A4 such as rifampin can decrease eszopiclone plasma levels.

Ramelteon (Rozerem)

Category: Sedative hypnotic.
Mechanism: Melatonin MT1 and MT2 agonist.
Indication: Insomnia, particularly sleep onset.
Preparation: 8 mg.
Dosage: 8 mg taken 30 minutes before bedtime.
Half-Life: 1-2.5 hours.
Clinical Guidelines: No associated tolerance or dependence. May decrease
testosterone levels and increase prolactin levels. Not a controlled substance.
Side Effects: Dizziness, fatigue, nausea, headache.
Drug Interactions: Strong CYP1A2 inhibitors, such as fluvoxamine, may increase
plasma levels of ramelteon by seventyfold and the two medications should not
be used together. Ramelteon plasma levels are also increased by CYP3A4
inhibitors such as ketoconazole and caution should be used in combination.
Strong inducers of cytochrome enzymes, such as rifampin, may decrease
efficacy of ramelteon. Ramelteon can potentiate the effect of other CNS
depressants, such as alcohol.

References, see page 115

Zaleplon (Sonata)

Category: Non-benzodiazepine hypnotic.
Mechanism: Binds to the GABA receptor, but is a non-benzodiazepine.
Indications: Insomnia.
Preparations: 5, 10 mg tablets.
Dosage: 10 mg qhs (5 mg for elderly).
Half-Life: 1 hr.
Clinical Guidelines: Zaleplon has a rapid onset of action. It is especially useful for initiating sleep and is not associated with dependence or withdrawal. Because of its short half-life, a repeat dose may be given. Not recommended if breast feeding.
Side Effects: Dizziness, dyspepsia, and diarrhea.
Drug Interactions: Potentiation of other CNS depressants (eg, alcohol). Higher serum levels have been reported in patients with hepatic insufficiency but not with moderate renal insufficiency. Cimetidine can increase serum levels.
Pregnancy: Category C.

Zolpidem (Ambien, Ambien CR)

Category: Non-benzodiazepine hypnotic.
Mechanism: Binds to the GABA receptor but is a non-benzodiazepine.
Indications: Insomnia.
Preparations: 5, 10 mg tablets.
Dosage: 10 mg qhs (5 mg for elderly).
Half-Life: 2-3 hrs.
Clinical Guidelines: Zolpidem has a rapid onset of action. It is especially useful for initiating sleep. Zolpidem is not associated with dependence or withdrawal. Ambien CR may be useful for patients that require a longer-acting sleep-aid. Although not recommended if breastfeeding, the American Academy of Pediatrics regards zolpidem as safe during lactation.
Side Effects: Dizziness, GI upset, nausea, vomiting. Anterograde amnesia and morning "hangover" occur at normal dosages. Rare reports of hallucinations.
Drug Interactions: Potentiation of other CNS depressants, such as alcohol. Higher serum levels reported in patients with hepatic insufficiency, but not with renal insufficiency.
Pregnancy: Category C.

References, see page 115.

Barbiturates

Barbiturate use has diminished since the introduction of benzodiazepines because of the lower therapeutic index and high abuse potential.

I. Indications
A. There are very few psychiatric indications for barbiturates because benzodiazepines are safer and equally effective. The phenobarbital challenge test is used to quantify sedative-hypnotic abuse in patients abusing multiple sedative hypnotics, including alcohol.
B. Given the availability of equally effective and safer benzodiazepines, it is difficult to justify the use of barbiturates.

II. Pharmacology
A. Barbiturates bind to barbiturate receptor sites, which are part of the GABA receptor. Barbiturate binding facilitates the action of GABA at the GABA receptor complex, resulting in inhibition.
B. Barbiturates induce hepatic microsomal enzymes and may reduce levels of other medications with hepatic metabolism.

III. Clinical Guidelines
A. Continued use of barbiturates for more than 3-4 weeks is associated with tolerance, dependence and a withdrawal syndrome.
  1. Tolerance develops to the sedative side effects. Cross-tolerance between barbiturates and other sedative hypnotic drugs, including alcohol, may develop.
  2. Withdrawal symptoms include: heightened anxiety, tremor, muscle twitching, sweating, insomnia, tachycardia, hypertension with postural hypotension and seizures.
  3. The severity of withdrawal is determined by the rate of decreasing serum level. Faster rates of decline are associated with more severe withdrawal.
B. Avoidance of an abstinence syndrome requires gradual tapering upon discontinuation. A long half-life benzodiazepine (eg, clonazepam) helps to reduce the severity of withdrawal.
C. Barbiturates should not be used in pregnancy. Infants born to habituated mothers may have respiratory depression at birth and will have withdrawal symptoms.

IV. Adverse Drug Reactions
A. The most common side effect is sedation and impaired concentration. Dizziness, ataxia and impaired fine motor coordination can also occur.
B. Barbiturates should not be used in patients with hepatic dysfunction because their metabolism will be impaired and toxicity may occur. Barbiturates are contraindicated in patients with acute intermittent porphyria because they may cause the production of porphyrins.

V. Drug Interactions
A. The concomitant use of benzodiazepines and CNS depressant agents, including sedative-hypnotics, will enhance sedation and increase the risk of respiratory depression. Alcohol use should be limited.
B. Barbiturates enhance the metabolism of a number of commonly used medications because they induce hepatic enzymes. Reduced effective-

ness of anticoagulants, tricyclic antidepressants, propranolol, carbamazepine, estrogen (oral contraceptives), corticosteroids, quinidine, and theophylline can occur.
C. The effect of barbiturates on phenytoin metabolism is unpredictable, phenytoin levels should be monitored. Valproate inhibits barbiturate metabolism.

Amobarbital

Preparations: 30, 50, 100 mg tablets; 65, 200 mg capsules; 250 mg/5 mL, 500 mg/5 mL solution (IM, IV).
Dosage:
  Sedation: 50-100 PO or IM.
  Hypnosis: 50-200 mg IV (max 400 mg/day).
Half-Life: 8-42 hrs.
Clinical Guidelines: Lorazepam has largely replaced the use of amobarbital for emergent control of psychotic agitation. The use of amobarbital in clinical diagnosis (Amytal interview) has also decreased and is not recommended.

Pentobarbital

Preparations: 50, 100 mg capsules.
Dosage: 200 mg PO.
Half-Life: 15-48 hrs.
Pentobarbital Challenge Test:
  A. The pentobarbital challenge test is a useful method of quantifying the daily intake of sedative hypnotics. Patients are given 200 mg orally and, after one hour, the level of intoxication is assessed. If there are no signs of intoxication, 100 mg is given, and the patient is reassessed after one hour.
  B. The procedure is repeated every two hours until signs of intoxication occur (nystagmus is the most sensitive sign and sleep is the most obvious sign). Maximum dose 600 mg. The dose required to show signs of intoxication is the equivalent dose to the daily habit of sedative hypnotics. Substitute a long half-life drug in divided doses and gradually taper by 10% per day.

References, see page 115.

Mood Stabilizers

Mood stabilizers are used for the treatment of mood episodes associated with bipolar and schizoaffective disorder as well as maintenance therapy. These agents are also used for the treatment of cyclothymia and unipolar depression.

Mood stabilizers can be helpful in the treatment of impulse control disorders, severe personality disorders, and behavioral disorders. Mood stabilizers include lithium and anticonvulsants. Atypical antipsychotics are indicated for treatment of mania and are being studied for their use in maintenance therapy.

Lithium Carbonate (Eskalith, Lithobid, Lithonate, Eskalith CR)

I. Indications
   A. Lithium is effective in the treatment of the acute manic phase of bipolar disorder as well as maintenance treatment of bipolar disorder. Lithium is more effective in the treatment of the manic episodes of bipolar disorder than in the depressed episodes. It is often necessary to add antidepressants to lithium when treating bipolar depressed patients.
   B. Lithium is also used clinically for schizoaffective disorder and severe cyclothymia.
   C. In depressed patients who have not responded to antidepressants, lithium augmentation may enhance response. Lithium augmentation may be a useful treatment strategy in some patients with schizophrenia who do not respond adequately to antipsychotics.
   D. Lithium may be helpful in treating borderline personality disorder and certain impulse control disorders, such as intermittent explosive disorder and behavioral disturbances.

II. Pharmacology
   A. Lithium may act by blocking inositol-1-phosphatase in neurons with subsequent interruption of the phosphatidylinositol second messenger system.
   B. Lithium is excreted by the kidneys. Impaired renal function or decreased fluid and salt intake can lead to toxicity. An age-related reduction in creatinine clearance will lead to reduced lithium clearance in the elderly. Lower doses and close monitoring are required in the elderly.
   C. Preparations
      1. Rapid absorption - Eskalith caps (300 mg), lithium carbonate caps and tabs (300 mg), Lithonate caps (300 mg), Lithotabs tabs (300 mg).
      2. Slow release - Lithobid tabs (300 mg), Eskalith CR (450 mg).
      3. Lithium citrate syrup: 8 mEq/5 mL (rapid absorption).
   D. Half-Life: 20 hrs.

III. Clinical Guidelines

A. Lithium is a first-line drug in the treatment of bipolar disorder. Valproate may also be used. Approximately 30% of patients with bipolar disorder will not respond to lithium.

B. **Pre-Lithium Work-Up:** Non-psychiatric causes of mood disorder or manic symptoms should be excluded before initiating lithium, including medical disorders, medications and substances of abuse. Screening laboratory studies include a basic chemistry panel, thyroid function tests, CBC, and an EKG in patients who are over 40 years old or with pre-existing cardiac disease. In females of childbearing age, pregnancy should be excluded.

IV. Dosage and Administration

A. Lithium is given in divided doses. Bid dosing with a slow-release formula is recommended. The starting dose for most adults is 300 mg bid-tid. The average dose rage is 900-2100 mg/day.

B. Single-daily dosing can be used if the daily dose is less than 1200 mg/day. Divided doses cause less GI upset and tremor.

C. Upward titration of lithium should occur until a serum level of 0.8-1.2 mEq/L is obtained. Some patients on long-term maintenance can be managed at lower serum levels between 0.5-0.8 mEq/L.

D. Serum lithium levels can be obtained after five days at any given dosage. Serum levels should be drawn 12 hours after the previous dose and are usually measured in the morning before the AM dose. Serum levels should be monitored weekly for the first 1-2 months, then biweekly for another 2 months. A patient who has been stable on lithium for a year can be monitored every 3-4 months.

E. **Therapeutic Response:** Therapeutic effect may take 4-6 weeks. True prophylactic effect may take >2 months.

F. **Pregnancy and Lactation:** Pregnancy category D. Lithium should not be administered to pregnant women in the first trimester when it is associated with an increased incidence of birth defects, especially Ebstein's anomaly. After the first trimester, lithium treatment may be initiated on a risk-benefit basis. Breastfeeding is contraindicated.

V. Adverse Drug Reactions

A. **Side Effects:** The most common side effects are GI distress, weight gain, fine tremor, and cognitive impairment ("fuzzy thinking"). Nausea, vomiting and tremor can be alleviated by dividing the dose, taking it with food or switching to a slow-release preparation. Small doses of propranolol (eg, 10 mg bid-tid) can reduce or eliminate tremor.

B. **Renal:** Polyuria with secondary polydipsia occurs in 20%. Lithium-induced diabetes insipidus may be treated with the diuretic, amiloride (5-10 mg/day). Renal function should be monitored.

C. **Thyroid:** Hypothyroidism may occur, which may be treated with levothyroxine. Monitor TSH several times per year.

D. **Cardiovascular:** Cardiovascular side effects include T-wave flattening or inversion and, rarely, arrhythmias, which usually require discontinuation. Edema may respond to spironolactone 50 mg/day or a reduction of the lithium dose.

E. **Dermatological:** Side effects include rash and acne, which may respond to dose reductions. Acne can be treated with benzoyl peroxide and topical antibiotics. Lithium can induce or exacerbate psoriasis, which usually resolves after discontinuation of lithium. Alopecia will also respond to discontinuation of lithium.

- **F. Hematologic:** A benign leukocytosis can occur with lithium. No treatment is indicated, but infection should be excluded.
- **G. Neurologic:** Muscle weakness, fasciculations, clonic movements, slurred speech and headaches have been reported. These symptoms may subside with time.
- **H. Lithium Toxicity**
    1. Toxicity may be caused by reduced fluid intake, increased fluid loss (excessive sweating) or reduced salt intake.
    2. Symptoms of lithium toxicity include nausea, vomiting, diarrhea, coarse tremor (in contrast to the fine tremor seen at therapeutic doses). Ataxia, headache, slurred speech, confusion, arrhythmias may also occur.
    3. Mild-to-moderate toxicity occurs at 1.5-2.0 mEq/L. Severe toxicity occurs at levels over 2.5 mEq/L. Death may occur at levels >4.0 mEq/L.

VI. Drug Interactions
- **A.** The most common cause of drug interactions is a change in the renal clearance of lithium.
- **B. Medications that decrease lithium levels include:**
    1. Xanthines (theophylline, aminophylline, caffeine).
    2. Increased dietary sodium and sodium bicarbonate (antacids).
    3. Carbonic anhydrase inhibitors (acetazolamide).
    4. Osmotic diuretics (mannitol).
- **C.** Medications that increase lithium levels and increase the risk of toxicity include diuretics, NSAIDS, COX-2 inhibitors, metronidazole and ACE-inhibitors.
- **D.** Neurotoxicity is a frequent consequence of lithium toxicity. Medications that will enhance the risk of lithium neurotoxicity include methyldopa, typical antipsychotics, carbamazepine, phenytoin and calcium channel blockers. Close monitoring for symptoms of neurotoxicity is recommended. Symptoms of neurotoxicity include tremor, disorientation, confusion, ataxia, and headaches.
- **E.** The action of neuromuscular-blocking agents, especially succinylcholine, will be prolonged by lithium. Prolonged recovery from electroconvulsive therapy, often requiring ventilatory assistance, may occur. Lithium should be discontinued prior to electroconvulsive therapy.

Olanzapine-Fluoxetine Combination (OFC, Symbyax)

I. Indications. FDA indication for bipolar depression.
II. Pharmacology
- **A.** Please refer to discussions of olanzapine and fluoxetine.
- **B.** Preparations (olanzapine/fluoxetine): 6/25, 6/50, 12/25, 12/50 mg capsules.
III. Clinical Guidelines
- **A.** The action or efficacy of OFC is equal to other atypical/SSRI combinations.

    B. Some patients may prefer taking only one tablet.
IV. Dosage and Administration
    A. Use of OFC is guided by the same principles that would apply when using olanzapine and fluoxetine separately.
V. Adverse Drug Reactions
    A. The most common side effects associated with OFC are asthenia, edema, increased appetite, somnolence, tremor, and weight gain.
    B. Please refer to the discussion of olanzapine and fluoxetine for further discussion of side effects.

References, see page 115.

Anticonvulsants

Anticonvulsants are primarily used for the treatment of bipolar disorder. Anticonvulsants are replacing lithium as a first-line treatment in acute mania and the long-term prophylaxis of mood episodes in bipolar disorder. One hypothesis underlying the prophylactic action of anticonvulsants in bipolar disorder is based on the theory of kindling, whereby repeated subthreshold stimulation of a neuron will eventually result in the spontaneous firing of the neuron.

Anticonvulsants are more effective than lithium in the treatment of rapid-cycling and mixed bipolar states. They are also useful for impulse control disorders, treatment-resistant depressive disorder, borderline personality disorder and other disorders with impulsive, unpredictable and/or aggressive behavior. Some newer anticonvulsants, such as pregabalin, tiagabine and levetiracetam are being studied for the treatment of bipolar disorder, but experience is very limited.

Carbamazepine (Tegretol)

I. Indications
   A. Carbamazepine is used for the treatment of the acute manic phase of bipolar disorder and for maintenance treatment of bipolar disorder. It may be used alone or in combination with lithium. It is more effective than lithium in treating rapid-cycling bipolar disorder and mixed episodes.
   B. Carbamazepine is more effective in the treatment and prophylaxis of manic episodes than the depressed episodes of bipolar disorder. When treating the depressed episode of bipolar disorder with an antidepressant, carbamazepine treatment should be monitored to prevent an anti-depressant-induced manic episode or rapid cycling.
   C. Carbamazepine is also used in the treatment of cyclothymia and schizo-affective disorder. It is used with antipsychotics and/or lithium in schizo-affective disorder.
   D. Carbamazepine augmentation of antipsychotic medication can be useful in patients with schizophrenia when there is inadequate response to antipsychotics alone. It is particularly helpful for aggressive or impulsive behavior.
   E. Carbamazepine may be helpful in treating certain impulse control disorders, such as those seen in patients with developmental disabilities. It may also be helpful to reduce symptoms of impulsivity and affective instability in patients with severe personality disorders. Carbamazepine may augment antidepressant treatment in depressed patients who are treatment-resistant.

II. Pharmacology
   A. The mechanism of action of carbamazepine in psychiatric disorders is unknown.
   B. Carbamazepine is metabolized by the liver (CYP3A4). The metabolites of carbamazepine are excreted renally. Carbamazepine will induce its own metabolism, and serum levels tend to decrease with time, requiring an

increase in the dosage. Initially, the half-life can be 25-65 hours. After several weeks, the serum half-life can decrease to 12-17 hours.

C. Preparations: 100, 200 mg tablets; 100 mg/5 mL oral suspension; 100 mg chewable tablets; 100, 200, 300, 400 mg extended-release tablets.

III. Clinical Guidelines

A. Pre-Carbamazepine Work-Up

1. Non-psychiatric causes of mood disorder or manic symptoms, including medical disorders, medications and substances of abuse should be excluded before beginning carbamazepine treatment.

2. Screening labs should include a basic chemistry panel, CBC, and an ECG in patients over 40 years old or with pre-existing cardiac disease. Pregnancy should be excluded in women of childbearing age.

B. Carbamazepine should not be given to patients with pre-existing liver, cardiac, or hematological disease. Carbamazepine is not recommended for patients with renal dysfunction because it has active metabolites that are renally excreted.

C. If carbamazepine is used in patients who have not responded to lithium, the carbamazepine should be added to the drug regimen with lithium. If the patient responds, the lithium should be discontinued.

D. Dosage and Administration

1. Starting dose is 200 mg bid. The average dose range is 600–1200 mg/day. The dosage should be reduced by one-half in the elderly.

2. A dosage increase, especially when initiating treatment, can cause a proportionally larger increase in serum level; therefore, the dosage should not be increased by more than 200 mg/day at a time.

3. Carbamazepine should be titrated to a serum level of 8-12 µg/mL. Serum carbamazepine levels should be obtained after five days at a given dosage. Serum levels should be drawn 12 hours after the previous dose, usually in the morning before the AM dose.

4. Serum levels should be monitored weekly for the first 1-2 months, then biweekly for another 2 months. Carbamazepine will induce its own metabolism, decreasing the serum level. The dosage may need to be increased in order to maintain a serum level within therapeutic range after initial stabilization.

5. A patient who has been stable on carbamazepine for a year can be monitored every 3-4 months. CBC and liver function, electrolytes and renal function should be checked after one month, then quarterly for the first year.

E. Therapeutic Response: Therapeutic effect may take 2-4 weeks.

F. Pregnancy and Lactation: Pregnancy category D. Carbamazepine is contraindicated during pregnancy or lactation. There is an association between use of carbamazepine in pregnancy and congenital malformations, including spina bifida.

IV. Adverse Drug Effects

A. Side Effects: The most common side effects are GI complaints (nausea, vomiting, constipation, diarrhea, loss of appetite) and CNS complaints (sedation, dizziness, ataxia, confusion). These can be prevented or significantly reduced by increasing the daily dosage slowly.

B. Hematological
1. Carbamazepine may cause life-threatening thrombocytopenia, agranulocytosis, and aplastic anemia in 0.005% of patients. Patients should contact their physician immediately if they have signs of infection (fever, sore throat) or bleeding abnormality (easy bruising, petechiae, pallor). A CBC should be drawn immediately. Carbamazepine should be discontinued if the WBC declines to less than 3000 mm^3, absolute neutrophil count <1500 mm^3 or platelet count decreases to <100,000 cells per mm^3.
2. Transient and minor decreases in blood cell indices can occur in the early phase of treatment and do not warrant discontinuation of carbamazepine.
C. Hepatic: Hepatitis and cholestatic jaundice may occur. The medication should be discontinued immediately.
D. Dermatological: Rash and urticaria are relatively common. Photosensitivity reactions may rarely occur. Potentially dangerous, but very rare, dermatological side effects include exfoliative dermatitis and toxic epidermal necrolysis (Stevens-Johnson syndrome), requiring immediate discontinuation of the drug.
E. Anticholinergic: Carbamazepine has mild anticholinergic activity and may exacerbate glaucoma and prostatic hypertrophy.
F. Cardiac: Uncommon side effects include AV conduction defects, arrhythmias, and congestive heart failure.
G. Metabolic/Endocrine: SIADH with hyponatremia has been reported.
H. Genitourinary: Urinary frequency, urinary retention, azotemia, renal failure and impotence are uncommon.
I. Toxicity: Signs of toxicity include confusion, stupor, motor restlessness, ataxia, dilated pupils, muscle twitching, tremor, athetoid movements, nystagmus, abnormal reflexes, oliguria, nausea and vomiting. Cardiac arrhythmias do not generally occur unless very large doses are ingested.

V. Drug Interactions
A. The following medications inhibit the metabolism of carbamazepine with resultant increase in serum levels and neurotoxicity:
1. Verapamil and diltiazem.
2. Danazol.
3. Erythromycin.
4. Fluoxetine.
5. Cimetidine (transient effect). Not seen with ranitidine or famotidine.
6. Isoniazid.
7. Ketoconazole.
8. Loratadine.
B. The following medications cause cytochrome P450 enzyme induction and decreased carbamazepine levels:
1. Rifampin.
2. Cisplatin.
C. Anticonvulsant Interactions with Carbamazepine
1. Phenobarbital will lower carbamazepine levels because of microsomal enzyme induction.
2. When phenytoin and carbamazepine are given at the same time, the levels of both drugs may be decreased.

3. Decreased ethosuximide levels because of cytochrome P450 enzyme induction.
4. Felbamate can decrease carbamazepine levels but increase the active metabolite of carbamazepine resulting in toxicities.
5. Lamotrigine and valproate can increase levels of the active metabolite. Patients may have signs of toxicity with normal carbamazepine levels. Carbamazepine will cause decreased valproate levels.

D. Carbamazepine will induce hepatic microsomal enzymes and enhance the metabolism (decrease serum levels and decrease the effectiveness) of the following medications:
1. Acetaminophen (may also enhance hepatotoxicity in overdose).
2. Clozapine and haloperidol.
3. Benzodiazepines (especially alprazolam, triazolam).
4. Oral contraceptives.
5. Corticosteroids.
6. Cyclosporine.
7. Doxycycline.
8. Mebendazole.
9. Methadone.
10. Theophylline (can also decrease carbamazepine levels).
11. Thyroid supplements (may mask compensatory increases in TSH).
12. Valproate.
13. Warfarin.

E. Diuretics should be used with caution because hyponatremia can occur with carbamazepine alone. A minimum 14-day washout should elapse before beginning an MAOI due to the molecular similarity between tricyclic antidepressants and carbamazepine.

Gabapentin (Neurontin)

I. Indications
A. Gabapentin is often used as an adjunctive agent in cyclic affective illness and other psychiatric conditions to alleviate anxiety and assist with sleep and low-grade irritability.
B. While initial studies with gabapentin showed promise in the treatment of cyclic affective illness, data do not currently indicate significant efficacy for this medication in monotherapy or as an adjunctive agent.

II. Pharmacology
A. Gabapentin is chemically related to the neurotransmitter GABA, but it does not act on GABA receptors. It is not converted into GABA, and it does not effect GABA metabolism or reuptake. The mechanism of action in psychiatric disorders is unknown.
B. Gabapentin is excreted renally in an unchanged state. Reduced clearance of gabapentin with age is largely caused by reduced renal function.
C. **Half-Life:** 5-7 hrs.
D. **Preparations:** 100, 300, 400 mg capsules; 600, 800 mg tablets; 250 mg/5 ml oral suspension.

III. Clinical Guidelines

A. Pre-Gabapentin Work-Up: Non-psychiatric causes of mood disorder or mood symptoms (mania and depression), including medical disorders, medications and substances of abuse, should be excluded before beginning gabapentin treatment. Renal function should be monitored. Pregnancy should be excluded in females of childbearing age.

B. Dosage and Administration

1. Starting dose is 300 mg qhs, then increasing by 300 mg each day. The average daily dose is between 900 and 1800 mg/day, but doses up to 2400 have been used.
2. Monitoring of serum levels is not necessary. There is no information available regarding a therapeutic window.
3. Significantly lower doses should be given to patients with impaired renal function or reduced creatinine clearance.

C. Therapeutic Response: 2-4 weeks

D. Pregnancy and Lactation: Pregnancy category C. There are no controlled studies in pregnant women. Gabapentin should be avoided during the first trimester. Mothers should be encouraged not to breast feed.

IV. Adverse Drug Reactions

A. Side Effects

1. The most common side effects are somnolence, fatigue, ataxia, nausea, vomiting and dizziness.
2. **Metabolic:** Weight gain, weight loss, edema.
3. **Cardiovascular:** Hypertension.
4. **GI:** Loss of appetite, increased appetite, dyspepsia, flatulence, gingivitis.
5. **Hematological:** Easy bruising.
6. **Musculoskeletal:** Arthralgia.
7. **CNS:** Nystagmus, tremor, diplopia, blurred vision.
8. **Psychiatric:** Anxiety, irritability, hostility, agitation, depression.

V. Drug Interactions

A. There are no interactions with other anticonvulsants.

B. Gabapentin has reduced absorption with antacids, and it should be taken at least 2 hours after antacid administration.

Lamotrigine (Lamictal)

I. Indications

A. Lamotrigine has efficacy in the treatment of bipolar depression as an adjunctive agent or as monotherapy. It has also been shown to decrease relapse to depression in stable bipolar patients compared to lithium. It is not effective against bipolar mania or rapid cycling. It is recommended that lamotrigine be used for maintenance treatment of bipolar disorder. It may be utilized for the treatment of bipolar depression.

B. Lamotrigine is more effective in depression compared to other mood stabilizers, prompting use in treatment-resistant unipolar depression. Controlled studies are currently underway.

II. Pharmacology

A. Lamotrigine may have an effect on sodium channels that modulate release of glutamate and aspartate. It also has a weak inhibitory effect on 5-HT$_3$ receptors.

B. Lamotrigine is hepatically metabolized via glucuronidation with subsequent renal excretion of the inactive glucuronide.

C. **Half-Life:** 25 hours.

D. **Preparations:** 25, 100, 150, 200 mg scored tablets; chewable tablets: 2, 5, 25 mg.

III. Clinical Guidelines

A. Non-psychiatric causes of mood disorder or mood symptoms (mania and depression), including medical disorders, medications and substances of abuse, should be excluded before beginning lamotrigine treatment.

B. Renal and hepatic function should be monitored. Pregnancy should be excluded in females of childbearing age.

C. **Dosage and Administration**

1. The initial dose is 25 mg/day, increased weekly to 50 mg/day, 100 mg/day, and then 200 mg/day.

2. In patients taking valproate, the dosage is 25 mg every other day for two weeks, then 25 mg per day for the next two weeks. In patients taking phenytoin, carbamazepine, phenobarbital or primidone without valproate, the dosage is 50 mg/day for two weeks, then 50 mg bid for the next two weeks. Average daily dose is 100-200 mg/day. Antidepressant effect may require up to 400 mg/day, which may be given in a divided dose.

3. Renal dysfunction does not markedly affect the half-life of lamotrigine. However, caution should be used when treating patients with renal disease since there is very little data in this population.

D. **Therapeutic Response:** Clinical effect: 2-4 weeks.

E. **Pregnancy and Lactation**

1. **Pregnancy Category C.** There are no controlled studies in pregnant women. Lamotrigine should be avoided during the first trimester.

2. Use after the first trimester is acceptable only if other agents are ineffective. Lamotrigine is excreted in breast milk. Mothers should not breast feed because the risks are unknown.

IV. Adverse Drug Effects

A. **Side Effects:** The most common side effects are dizziness, sedation, headache, diplopia, ataxia, and decreased coordination.

B. **Dermatological:** The side effect most likely to cause discontinuation of the drug is rash (10% incidence). Severe Stevens-Johnson syndrome (toxic epidermal necrolysis) can occur. Rash is most likely to occur in the first 4-6 weeks.

C. **Metabolic:** Weight gain.

D. **GI:** Nausea and vomiting.

E. **Psychiatric:** Agitation, irritability anxiety, depression and mania.

V. Drug Interactions

A. Carbamazepine-induced enzyme induction will enhance lamotrigine metabolism, resulting in lower levels than expected. Lamotrigine will increase the levels of and metabolites of carbamazepine.

B. Valproate will increase lamotrigine levels (as much as two times), and lamotrigine will decrease valproate levels slightly.

C. Phenobarbital-induced enzyme induction will lower lamotrigine levels.

D. Phenytoin will decrease lamotrigine levels.

E. No interaction with lithium has been reported.

F. Alcohol may enhance the side effects of lamotrigine.

G. Lamotrigine can be used with MAOIs.

Oxcarbazepine (Trileptal)

I. Indications

    A. Oxcarbazepine has been studied for use in mood disorders. It may be as effective as carbamazepine for bipolar disorder and better tolerated.

II. Pharmacology

    A. Chemically similar to carbamazepine.

    B. The mechanism of action of oxcarbazepine is unknown, but it is thought to exert its anticonvulsant properties by blockade of voltage-sensitive sodium channels. The active component is the 10-monohydroxy metabolite.

    C. Preparations: 150, 300, 600 mg scored tablets; 300 mg/5 mL oral suspension.

III. Clinical Guidelines

    A. Starting dose is 300 mg PO bid, increased by 600 mg each week to maintenance dose of 1200-2400 mg/day.

    B. Oxcarbazepine has fewer drug interactions than carbamazepine and is not associated with neutropenia.

    C. Patients switched from carbamazepine typically require 1.5 times the dose of oxcarbazepine.

    D. Pregnancy: Category C.

IV. Adverse Drug Reactions

    A. Somnolence, dizziness, diplopia, ataxia, nausea, vomiting and rash.

    B. Oxcarbazepine appears to have a lower incidence of hematologic, dermatologic (Stevens-Johnson syndrome), and hepatic toxicity compared to carbamazepine.

V. Drug Interactions

    A. Oxcarbazepine inhibits CYP2C19 and induces CYP3A4/5.

    B. Serum concentration of oxcarbazepine can be reduced by CYP450 inducers (phenobarbital, carbamazepine).

Pregabalin (Lyrica)

I. Indications

    A. Pregabalin has been studied for use in general anxiety disorder. A number of controlled trials support its efficacy. There is little evidence to support its use in bipolar disorder.

II. Pharmacology

    A. Pregabalin has structural similarities to gabapentin.

    B. Pregabalin blocks voltage dependent calcium channels.

III. Clinical Guidelines
    A. Starting dose is 50 mg PO tid or 75 mg PO bid, increased after one week
    to 300 mg/day. Maintenance dose is 150-600 mg/day.

IV. Adverse Drug Reactions
    A. Dizziness and drowsiness are the most common side effects; less
    common are blurred vision, ataxia, dysarthria, tremors, weight gain, dry
    mouth, edema, and constipation.
    B. The FDA considers pregabalin to have some abuse liability; therefore, it
    is schedule V.

V. Drug Interactions
    A. Minimal drug interactions, no protein binding.
    B. Excreted primarily unchanged by the kidneys.

Tiagabine (Gabitril)

I. Indications
    A. Tiagabine has no proven effectiveness in the treatment of psychiatric
    disorders to date. Preliminary work suggests that it may be effective in
    the treatment of anxiety.

II. Pharmacology
    A. The mechanism of action is unknown, but it may enhance the action of
    GABA in the CNS.
    B. Tiagabine is metabolized via the CYP3A4 enzyme system.
    C. Half-Life: 7-9 hours.
    D. Preparations: 2, 4, 12, 16, 20 mg tablets.

III. Clinical Guidelines
    A. Initial dose: 4 mg PO q day, increase by 4-8 mg/week in divided doses
    up to 56 mg/day. Total daily dosages greater than 32 mg should be
    divided into three or four doses per day.
    B. Reduced dosages should be used in patients with hepatic disease or
    impairment.
    C. Pregnancy and Lactation: Category C.

IV. Adverse Drug Reactions
    A. The most common side effects are dizziness, fatigue, somnolence,
    nausea, irritability, tremor, abdominal pain, and decreased concentration.
    B. Generalized weakness may occur. Weakness is usually alleviated by
    dose reduction or discontinuation of medication.

V. Drug Interactions
    A. CYP 450 inducers will significantly decrease the serum concentration of
    tiagabine.
    B. Tiagabine can cause a slight (10%) decrease in serum valproate levels.
    C. CYP3A4 inhibitors can increase the serum concentration of tiagabine.

Topiramate (Topamax)

I. Indications
  A. Studies do not support the effectiveness of topiramate in the treatment of bipolar disorder. It is sometimes used as adjunctive treatment to promote weight loss.
  B. Other open label clinical studies have suggested potential effectiveness of topiramate in impulse control disorders, bulimia, migraine, alcohol craving, and post traumatic stress disorder.

II. Pharmacology
  A. The mechanism of action is unknown.
  B. Topiramate is not extensively metabolized and is mostly excreted unchanged in the urine.
  C. **Half-Life:** Approximately 21 hours.
  D. **Preparations:** 25, 100 and 200 mg tablets; 15 and 25 mg sprinkle capsules.

III. Clinical Guidelines
  A. Non-psychiatric causes of mood disorder or mood symptoms (mania and depression), including medical disorders, medications and substances of abuse should be excluded before beginning topiramate treatment.
  B. Renal and hepatic function should be monitored. Pregnancy should be excluded in females of childbearing age.
  C. Topiramate is associated with appetite suppression and possible weight loss, which may be desirable in some patients. Minimal hepatic metabolism may make it preferable over other anticonvulsants.
  D. **Dosage and Administration**
    1. **Initial dose:** 25-50 mg qhs, then increase in 25-50 mg increments per week up to 400 mg/day in divided doses.
    2. Patients with renal impairment should take 1/2 the recommended dose.
    3. No adjustments are necessary for the elderly.
  E. **Pregnancy and Lactation:** Category C.

IV. Adverse Effects
  A. The most common side effects are fatigue, somnolence, dizziness, nausea, anorexia, decreased concentration, ataxia, anxiety, and paresthesias. Appetite suppression and weight loss may be welcome side effects.
  B. Topiramate can cause hyperchloremic, non-anion gap metabolic acidosis. Use in patients with renal disease, severe respiratory disorders, diarrhea and ketogenic diets can result in lower bicarbonate levels. There is a small risk (1%) of nephrolithiasis. This can be minimized by maintaining good hydration.

V. Drug Interactions
  A. Carbamazepine-induced enzyme induction will reduce topiramate levels.
  B. When given with valproic acid, both topiramate and valproate levels may decrease.
  C. When given with phenytoin, topiramate levels will decrease and phenytoin levels increase.
  D. Concomitant use of phenobarbital can decrease topiramate levels.
  E. Concomitant use of acetazolamide will increase the risk of nephrolithiasis and should be avoided.

F. Topiramate may decrease serum digoxin levels. Topiramate may reduce the effectiveness of oral contraceptives by reducing estrogen levels.

Valproic Acid (Depakene) and Divalproex (Depakote, Depakote ER)

I. Indications
A. Valproate may be used with lithium or alone in bipolar disorder and schizoaffective disorder.
B. Valproate is more effective in rapid cycling and mixed episode bipolar disorder than lithium.
C. Recent evidence suggests that valproate may be more effective in treating depressive episodes compared to lithium and carbamazepine. However, it remains more effective in the treatment and prophylaxis of manic episodes than the depressed episodes of bipolar disorder.
D. Valproate augmentation may be a useful treatment strategy in patients with schizophrenia who have not responded adequately to antipsychotics alone. Valproate is particularly helpful in patients with aggressive or impulsive behavior.
E. There have been reports that valproate may be helpful in treating certain impulse control disorders, such as intermittent explosive disorder and aggressive, impulsive behavior in patients with developmental disabilities. Valproate may also be helpful to reduce symptoms of impulsivity and affective instability in patients with severe personality disorders.

II. Psychopharmacology
A. Valproate may also affect neuronal signal transduction though actions on protein kinase C. It is unknown if these mechanisms underlie the effectiveness of valproate in psychiatric disorders.
B. The average half-life is 8-10 hours, making bid-tid dosing necessary.
C. **Pharmacokinetics and Metabolism of Valproate**
   1. Valproate is metabolized by the liver by the mitochondrial beta-oxidation, glucuronidation and the P450 microsomal system. Unlike many other psychotropic medications, cytochrome P450 is relatively unimportant in valproate metabolism, and medications that affect P450 have little effect on valproate serum levels.
   2. Serum levels can be helpful to establish minimum dosages at the low end of the therapeutic range, but at higher levels, it is more important to monitor clinical symptoms of toxicity and side effects.
   3. Valproate is highly protein bound and, at higher concentrations, serum proteins become saturated, resulting in more unbound drug being available. This enhances the metabolism of the drug and lowers the serum concentration.
   4. Decreased protein binding (higher serum levels) is seen in the elderly and in patients with hepatic and renal disease. These patients are at greater risk for toxicity.
D. **Preparations**: Valproic acid – 250 mg capsules; 250 mg/5 mL oral susp. Divalproex (enteric coated) – 125 mg, 250 mg, 500 mg tablets. Extended release (Depakote ER) – 250, 500 mg tablets Sprinkle capsules – 125mg.

III. **Clinical Guidelines**
   A. Valproate may be used as a first-line drug in the treatment of bipolar disorder, especially in patients with rapid cycling bipolar disorder or mixed mood episode.
   B. Valproate should not be given to patients with pre-existing hepatic or hematological disease.
   C. **Pre-Valproate Work-Up**
      1. Non-psychiatric causes of mood disorder or manic symptoms, including medical disorders, medications and substances of abuse, should be excluded before beginning valproate treatment.
      2. Screening laboratory exams should include liver function tests and a CBC. In females of childbearing age, pregnancy should be excluded.
   D. **Dosage and Administration**
      1. Initiation of treatment begins with 20 mg/kg/day or 500 mg tid or 750 mg bid, then titrating up or down, depending on the serum level. The average daily dose is between 1500 and 2500 mg/day. The extended-release formulation allows once-daily dosing, and the bioavailability is 80-90% compared to Depakote. Elderly patients will require doses nearly half that of younger adults.
      2. A serum level of 50-125 µg/mL is usually adequate for symptom relief. Serum levels in the low range are more accurate and more clinically useful compared to the high end of the therapeutic range. Patients can often tolerate levels up to 150 µg/mL.
      3. Serum valproate levels can be obtained after 3 days at any given dosage. Serum levels should be drawn 12 hours after the previous dose and are usually done in the morning before the AM dose.
      4. Serum levels should be monitored weekly for the first 1-2 months, then biweekly for another 2 months. A patient who has been stable for a year can be monitored every 3-4 months. CBC and liver function tests should be drawn after one month, then quarterly for the first year.
   E. **Therapeutic Response:** Therapeutic effect may take 2-4 weeks.
   F. **Pregnancy and Lactation:** Pregnancy category D. Valproate should not be used in pregnancy or breastfeeding. An increased incidence of neural tube defects and other birth defects has been reported. Fatal clotting abnormalities and hepatic failure have occurred in infants.
IV. **Adverse Drug Reactions**
   A. **Side Effects:** The most common side effects are sedation, dizziness, nausea and vomiting (divalproex has lower incidence of GI side effects). GI side effects tend to decrease over time, especially if the drug is taken with food.
   B. **Pancreatitis:** A rare but serious adverse effect is pancreatitis, usually occurring early in treatment.
   C. **Hepatic**
      1. Hepatitis, which can be fatal, occurs in 0.0005% of patients. It is most common in children. Symptoms include lethargy, malaise, vomiting, loss of appetite, jaundice and weakness, usually occurring in the first 6 months of treatment. Valproate should be discontinued immediately if hepatitis is suspected.
      2. A transient early increase in liver enzymes may occur in up to 25% of patients, but the increase does not predict the development of hepatitis.

Close monitoring of liver enzymes is important to distinguish the benign temporary increase in hepatic enzymes from more dangerous hepatitis.
   D. **Hematological:** Thrombocytopenia and platelet dysfunction can occur with secondary bleeding abnormalities.
   E. **Neurological:** Tremor, ataxia, headache, insomnia, agitation.
   F. **Other GI Side Effects:** Changes in appetite and weight, diarrhea, constipation.
   G. **Dermatological:** Alopecia, maculopapular rash.
   H. **Overdose:** Symptoms of toxicity/overdose include somnolence, heart block and coma.
   I. **Urea Cycle Disorders:** Hyperammonemic encephalopathy, sometimes fatal, can occur in patients with rare urea cycle disorders. Urea cycle disorders, such as ornithine transcarbamlyase deficiency.

V. Drug Interactions
   A. The following medications inhibit the metabolism of valproate with resultant increases in serum levels and increased potential for toxicity:
      1. Aspirin inhibits metabolism and decreases bound fraction.
      2. Felbamate.
   B. Rifampin will increase valproate clearance and result in decreased serum concentrations.
   C. **Anticonvulsant Interactions**
      1. Phenobarbital causes non-P450 enzyme induction and lowers valproate levels. Valproate inhibits phenobarbital metabolism.
      2. Phenytoin causes non-P450 enzyme induction and lowers valproate levels. Levels of both drugs should be monitored.
      3. Carbamazepine causes non-P450 enzyme induction and lowers valproate levels. Valproate may not affect carbamazepine levels but will increase serum levels of the active metabolite. Patients should be monitored for symptoms of carbamazepine toxicity.
      4. Valproate inhibits the metabolism of lamotrigine and ethosuximide.
      5. The combination of valproate and clonazepam has been reported to cause absence seizures.
   D. **Other Interactions**
      1. Valproate inhibits the metabolism of diazepam, amitriptyline, and nortriptyline, resulting in increased levels.
      2. Valproate inhibits the metabolism of AZT.
      3. Valproate can displace warfarin from protein binding. Careful monitoring of clotting times is recommended.

References, see page 115.

Psychostimulants

Dextroamphetamine (Dexedrine, Dextrostat)

I. Indications
  A. Dextroamphetamine has been approved for the treatment of narcolepsy and Attention-Deficit Hyperactivity Disorder (ADHD). It is used in the treatment of ADHD in children and adults.
  B. Dextroamphetamine is used as an adjunct to antidepressants in patients who have had an inadequate response to antidepressants. It has also been used effectively in depressed medically ill or elderly patients who have not been able to tolerate antidepressants.

II. Pharmacology
  A. Dextroamphetamine is the d-isomer of amphetamine. It is a centrally acting sympathomimetic amine and causes the release of norepinephrine from neurons. At higher doses, it will also cause dopamine and serotonin release. It inhibits CNS monoamine oxidase activity.
  B. Peripheral effects include increased blood pressure and pulse, respiratory stimulation, mydriasis, and weak bronchodilation.
  C. **Preparations:** Dextroamphetamine sulfate (Dexedrine) 5, 10 mg tabs; elixir 5 mg/5 mL; Dexedrine Spansule (sustained release) 5, 10, 15 mg caps; dextroamphetamine sulfate (Dextrostat) 5, 10 mg scored tabs.
  D. **Half-Life:** 8-12 hrs.

III. Clinical Guidelines
  A. Dextroamphetamine is a schedule II controlled substance, requiring a triplicate prescription. Dextroamphetamine has a high potential for abuse because it increases energy and productivity. Tolerance and intense psychological dependence develop.
  B. Symptoms upon discontinuation may include fatigue and depression. Chronic users can become suicidal upon abrupt cessation of the drug.
  C. **Pre-Dextroamphetamine Work-Up**
   1. Blood pressure and general cardiac status should be evaluated prior to initiating dextroamphetamine.
   2. Since dextroamphetamine can precipitate tics and Tourette' syndrome, careful screening for movement disorders should be completed prior to beginning treatment.
  D. Dextroamphetamine is contraindicated in patients with hypertension, hyperthyroidism, cardiac disease, or glaucoma. It is not recommended for psychotic patients or patients with a history of substance abuse.
  E. **Dosage and Administration**
   1. **Attention-Deficit Hyperactivity Disorder:** The initial dosage is 2.5-5.0 mg bid-tid. Increase gradually in divided doses (7 am, 11 am or noon, 3 pm) until optimal response. The maximum total daily dose is 1.0 mg/kg/day for children or 40 mg/day for adults. The spansule preparation can be given bid.
   2. **Depression (medically ill):** 5-20 mg/day.
   3. **Narcolepsy:** 10-60 mg/day in divided doses.

    4. Children under the age of 3 should not be given dextroamphetamine.
  F. Weight and growth should be monitored in all children. Weight loss and growth delay are reasons to discontinue medication.
  G. Pregnancy and Lactation: Pregnancy category C. There is an increased risk of premature delivery and low birth weight in infants born to mothers using amphetamines. Dextroamphetamine is contraindicated in pregnancy or lactation.

IV. Adverse Drug Reactions
  A. Side Effects: The most common side effects are psychomotor agitation, insomnia, loss of appetite, and dry mouth. Tolerance to loss of appetite tends to develop. Effect on sleep can be reduced by not giving the drug after 12 pm.
  B. Cardiovascular: Palpitations, tachycardia, increased blood pressure
  C. CNS: Dizziness, euphoria, tremor, precipitation of tics, Tourette's syndrome, and, rarely, psychosis.
  D. GI: Anorexia and weight loss, diarrhea, constipation.
  E. Growth inhibition: Chronic administration of psychostimulants has been associated with growth delay in children. Growth should be monitored.
  F. Toxicity/Overdose: Symptoms include insomnia, irritability, hostility, psychomotor agitation, psychosis with paranoid features, hypertension, tachycardia, sweating, hyperreflexia, tachypnea. At very high doses, patients can present with arrhythmias, nausea, vomiting, circulatory collapse, seizures and coma.

V. Drug Interactions
  A. High blood levels of propoxyphene can enhance the CNS stimulatory effects of dextroamphetamine, causing seizures and death
  B. Dextroamphetamine will enhance the activity of tricyclic and tetracyclic antidepressants, and will also potentiate their cardiovascular effects.
  C. Dextroamphetamine may antagonize the effects of antihypertensives.
  D. Typical antipsychotics and lithium can inhibit the CNS stimulatory effects of dextroamphetamine.
  E. Fatal reactions are likely if psychostimulants are given with MAOIs. Hypertensive crisis and seizures may occur. MAOIs should be discontinued for at least 14 days prior to the initiation of dextroamphetamine.
  F. Dextroamphetamine will delay the absorption of ethosuximide, phenobarbital and phenytoin.

Dextroamphetamine and Amphetamine (Adderall, Adderall XR)

I. Indications
    A. Adderall is indicated for the treatment of Attention-Deficit Hyperactivity Disorder (ADHD) and Narcolepsy.

II. Pharmacology
    A. Adderall is a combination of dextroamphetamine and amphetamine. The combination has a similar pharmacology to Dexedrine.

    B. Preparations: Adderall 5, 7.5, 10, 12.5, 15, 20, 30 mg tablets; Adderall XR 5, 10, 15, 20, 25, 30 mg capsules

    C. Dosing: 5-10 mg/day. The average dose is 20-30 mg/day for ADHD and 5-60 mg for narcolepsy. Maximum dose is 40 mg for children and 60 mg for adults.

III. Clinical Guidelines
    A. Adderall is a schedule II controlled substance, requiring a triplicate prescription. Adderall has a high potential for abuse because it increases energy and productivity. Tolerance and intense psychological dependence develop.

    B. Symptoms upon discontinuation may include fatigue and depression. Chronic users can become suicidal upon abrupt cessation of the drug.

    C. Pre-Adderall Work-Up
        1. Blood pressure should be evaluated prior to initiating dextroamphetamine.
        2. Since Adderall can precipitate tics and Tourette's syndrome, screening for movement disorders should be completed prior to beginning treatment.

    D. Adderall is contraindicated in patients with hypertension, hyperthyroidism, cardiac disease or glaucoma. It is not recommended for psychotic patients or patients with a history of substance abuse.

    E. Weight and growth should be monitored in all children. Weight loss and growth delay are reasons to discontinue medication.

    F. Pregnancy and Lactation: Pregnancy category C. There is an increased risk of premature delivery and low birth weight in infants born to mothers using amphetamines. Adderall is contraindicated in pregnancy and lactation.

IV. Adverse Drug Reactions
    A. Side Effects: The most common side effects are psychomotor agitation, insomnia, loss of appetite, and dry mouth. Tolerance to loss of appetite tends to develop. Effects on sleep can be reduced by not giving the drug after 12 pm.

    B. Cardiovascular: Palpitations, tachycardia, increased blood pressure.

    C. CNS: Dizziness, euphoria, tremor, precipitation of tics, Tourette's syndrome, and, rarely, psychosis.

    D. GI: Anorexia, weight loss, diarrhea, constipation.

    E. Growth inhibition: Chronic administration of psychostimulants has been associated with growth delay in children. Growth should be monitored during treatment.

    F. Toxicity/Overdose: Symptoms include insomnia, irritability, hostility, psychomotor agitation, psychosis with paranoid features, hypertension, tachycardia, sweating, hyperreflexia, tachypnea. At very high doses, patients can present with arrhythmias, nausea, vomiting, circulatory collapse, seizures and coma.

V. Drug Interactions

    A. High blood levels of propoxyphene can enhance the CNS stimulatory effects of Adderall, causing seizures and death.

    B. Adderall will enhance the activity of tricyclic and tetracyclic antidepressants and will also potentiate their cardiovascular effects.

    C. Typical antipsychotics and lithium can inhibit the CNS stimulatory effects of Adderall and other amphetamine preparations.

    D. Fatal reactions are likely if psychostimulants are given with MAOIs. Hypertensive crisis or seizures may occur. MAOIs should be discontinued for at least 14 days prior to the initiation of Adderall.

    E. Adderall will delay the absorption of the ethosuximide, phenobarbital and phenytoin.

Methylphenidate (Ritalin, Ritalin SR, Ritalin LA, Concerta, Metadate ER, Metadate CD, Focalin, Focalin XR, Methylin, Methylin ER, Attenade, Daytrana)

I. Indications

    A. Methylphenidate is the most commonly used medication in the treatment of Attention-Deficit Hyperactivity Disorder (ADHD) in children and adults. It is also used in the treatment of narcolepsy.

    B. Methylphenidate is also used for depression as an adjunct to antidepressants in patients who have an inadequate response to antidepressants. It has also been used effectively in depressed, medically ill or elderly patients who have not been able to tolerate antidepressants.

II. Pharmacology

    A. Methylphenidate is a CNS stimulant, which is chemically related to amphetamine. Methylphenidate is metabolized by hydroxylation and then renally excreted.

    B. Preparations: 5, 10, 20 mg tabs; sustained-release (SR) 20 mg tabs; long-acting (LA) 20, 30 and 40 mg capsules. The SR tablet should be swallowed whole and not crushed or chewed. Concerta: 18, 27, 36 and 54 mg extended-release tablets. Metadate CD: 10, 20 and 30 mg capsules. Metadate ER: 10 and 20 mg tabs. Focalin 2.5, 5, 10 mg tabs. Focalin XR: 5, 10, 20 mg capsules. Methylin: 5, 10, 20 mg tablets. Methylin ER: 10 and 20 mg tablets. Daytrana Patch 10 mg/9hrs, 15 mg/9hrs, 20 mg/9hrs, 30 mg/9hrs.

    C. Half-Life: 3-4 hrs; 6-8 hrs for sustained release.

III. Clinical Guidelines

A. Methylphenidate is a schedule II controlled substance, requiring a triplicate prescription. It has a high potential for abuse. Tolerance and psychological dependence can develop.

B. Symptoms upon discontinuation may include severe fatigue and depression. Chronic users can become suicidal upon abrupt cessation of the drug.

C. Pre-Methylphenidate Work-Up
   1. Blood pressure should be evaluated prior to initiating treatment. The cardiac risk with methylphenidate is less than that for dextroamphetamine.
   2. Leukopenia, anemia and elevated liver enzymes have been reported; therefore, baseline and periodic blood counts and liver function tests are recommended.
   3. Since methylphenidate can precipitate tics and Tourette's syndrome, screening for movement disorders should be completed prior to beginning treatment.

D. Patients with hypertension, seizure disorder and symptomatic cardiac disease should not take methylphenidate. Methylphenidate is not recommended for psychotic patients or patients with a history of substance abuse.

E. Weight and growth should be monitored in children. Weight loss and growth failure are reasons to discontinue medication.

F. Dosage and Administration
   1. **Attention-Deficit Hyperactivity Disorder**
      a. Initiate with 5 mg bid. Increase by 5-10 mg each week until optimal response achieved. Usual dose: 10-60 mg/day (max 2.0 mg/kg/day). The initial dosage of Concerta is 18 mg/day, with an average dose of 18-54 mg/day.
      b. Ritalin LA releases an immediate dose of methylphenidate with a second release (via enteric-coated, delayed-release beads) four hours later. The recommended starting dosage of Ritalin LA is 20 mg, titrated by 10 mg per week as needed up to 60 mg/day.
      c. Focalin is the d-isomer (dexmethylphenidate) of methylphenidate. The recommended conversion is half the dose of racemic methylphenidate.
      d. Daytrana Patch should be applied 2 hours before the effect is needed and removed after 9 hours. Dose may be titrated between 10 and 30 mg per day.
   2. **Depression (medically ill):** 10-20 mg/day.
   3. **Augmentation of Antidepressant:** 10-40 mg/day.
   4. Safety and efficacy in children under the age of 6 has not been established.

G. Pregnancy and Lactation: Methylphenidate is contraindicated in pregnant or lactating women.

IV. Adverse Drug Reactions

A. Side Effects: The most common side effects are nervousness and insomnia, which these can be reduced by decreasing dose.

B. Cardiovascular: Hypertension, tachycardia, arrhythmias.

    C. **CNS:** Dizziness, euphoria, tremor, headache, precipitation of tics and Tourette's syndrome and, rarely, psychosis.

    D. **GI:** Decreased appetite, weight loss. Case reports of elevated liver enzymes and liver failure.

    E. **Hematological:** Leukopenia and anemia have been reported.

    F. **Growth inhibition:** Chronic administration of psychostimulants has been associated with growth delay in children. Growth should be monitored during treatment.

    G. **Toxicity/Overdose:** Symptoms include agitation, tremors, hyperreflexia, confusion, psychosis, psychomotor agitation, tachycardia, sweating and hypertension. At very high doses, patients can present with seizures, arrhythmias, and coma.

V. **Drug Interactions**

    A. Methylphenidate may antagonize the effects of antihypertensives.

    B. Methylphenidate decreases the metabolism and increases the level of the following medications:

        1. Tricyclic and tetracyclic antidepressants.

        2. Warfarin.

        3. Phenytoin, phenobarbital and primidone.

        4. Phenylbutazone.

    C. **Sudden Death:** There have been case reports of sudden cardiac death when methylphenidate and clonidine have been used together.

Atomoxetine (Strattera)

I. **Indications**

    A. Attention-Deficit Hyperactivity Disorder in both children and adults.

    B. Clinical trials in depressed patients showed that the drug was ineffective for depression, but there have been anecdotal reports suggesting that it may be useful as an adjunctive treatment in depression and schizophrenia because of improved cognition.

II. **Pharmacology**

    A. Atomoxetine is a presynaptic norepinephrine transporter inhibitor, which causes enhancement of noradrenergic function. Atomoxetine is not considered a psychostimulant and is not a controlled substance.

    B. Atomoxetine may be equally effective as methlphenidate, but it has a lower incidence of appetite suppression and insomnia.

    C. **Metabolism:** Atomoxetine is metabolized via the CYP2D6 enzyme.

    D. **Half-Life:** Approximately 4 hours.

    E. **Preparations:** 10, 18, 25, 40, and 60 mg capsules.

    F. **Dosage**

        1. In children (<70 kg) the dose should be initiated at 0.5 mg/kg and increased to a target dose of 1.2 mg/kg/day. The dose should not exceed 1.4 mg/kg or 100 mg/day, whichever is less.

        2. In adults (>70 kg), the initial dose is 40 mg/day, which is increased to 80 mg/day. Dose can be increased to 100 mg/day after 2-4 weeks. The dose should not exceed 100 mg.

   3. The dose can be given in the morning or divided between morning and late afternoon.

III. Clinical Guidelines

   A. Dividing the dose may reduce some side effects.

   B. Dose reductions are necessary in the presence of moderate hepatic insufficiency.

   C. Atomoxetine should not be used within 2 weeks of discontinuation of an MAOI.

   D. Atomoxetine should be avoided in patients with narrow angle glaucoma, and it should be used with caution in patients with tachycardia, hypertension or cardiovascular disease.

   E. Atomoxetine can be discontinued without a taper.

   F. Pregnancy and Lactation: Category C.

IV. Adverse Drug Reactions

   A. Hepatic Injury: Atomoxetine can cause severe liver injury in rare cases. Lab testing should be performed if any signs of liver dysfunction occur, such as dark urine, or pruritis.

   B. Suicidal Ideation: Atomoxetine increased the risk of suicidal ideation in studies of children and adolescents with ADHD. The average risk of suicidal ideation was 0.4% compared to none with placebo. A black box warning has been issued by the FDA.

   C. Cardiovascular: Increased blood pressure and heart rate (similar to those seen with conventional psychostimulants).

   D. Gastrointestinal: Anorexia, weight loss, nausea, abdominal pain.

   E. Miscellaneous: Fatigue, dry mouth, constipation, urinary hesitancy and erectile dysfunction.

V. Drug Interactions:
Individuals with decreased activity of the CYP2D6 enzyme (5-10% of the population) or who are taking CYP2D6 inhibitors (eg, fluoxetine, paroxetine) will have fivefold greater plasma levels and the drug will have a longer half-life (24 hours).

Modafinil (Provigil)

I. Indications

   A. Excessive Daytime Sleepiness associated with Narcolepsy.

   B. There is anecdotal evidence for the use of modafinil as adjunctive treatment in depression, for negative symptoms of schizophrenia and for cognitive alertness in dementia. Some evidence exists for the effectiveness of modafinil (300 mg qam) for ADHD.

II. Pharmacology

   A. Modafinil is metabolized by the liver (3A4 enzyme). 3A4 inhibitors or inducers may affect the metabolism of modafinil. Absorption is delayed by food.

   B. Preparations: 100 and 200 mg tablets.

   C. Half-Life: 15 hrs.

III. Clinical Guidelines

A. Modafinil is generally well tolerated, with little effect on nighttime sleep. It has less side effects and less abuse potential than amphetamine-like stimulants.

B. Limited data suggests that modafinil may be useful in antidepressant augmentation or for improving fatigue in illnesses such as chronic fatigue syndrome.

C. **Dosage and Administration:** Initial dosage is 200 mg/day (8 AM). Elderly and patients with hepatic impairment require a lower dose. Some patients may benefit from a mid-afternoon dose (100-200 mg). The maximum recommended daily dose is 400 mg/day.

D. **Pregnancy and Lactation:** Category C.

IV. Adverse Drug Reactions

A. **Side Effects:** The most common side effects are headache, nausea, diarrhea, and anorexia. Anxiety, nervousness, and insomnia have been reported but are less frequent, compared to methylphenidate.

B. **Toxicity/Overdose:** Symptoms include nausea, diarrhea, palpitations, tremor, sleep disturbance, irritability, aggressiveness, and confusion.

V. Drug Interactions.
Potential interactions exist with inducers, substrates, or inhibitors of the 3A4 hepatic enzyme. Other potential interactions may exist with the 2D6 and 2C19 enzymes. Use with MAOIs should be avoided.

References, see page 115.

Substance Dependence

Management of Substance Dependence

I. **Management of Substance Dependence**

  A. **Alcohol Dependence/Withdrawal:** Prolonged use of large amounts of alcohol leads to dependence and withdrawal upon discontinuation. Withdrawal can be fatal if the patient develops delirium tremens and subsequent electrolyte abnormalities or cardiac arrhythmias. Benzodiazepines, such as lorazepam and chlordiazepoxide, are used to prevent withdrawal symptoms.

  B. **Alcohol Relapse:** Disulfiram and naltrexone are used to help prevent relapse once a patient has been detoxified. These agents should be used in conjunction with a behavior modification program, such as Alcoholics Anonymous. Acamprosate is effective in maintaining abstinence but should be used as part of a comprehensive psychosocial program. Some early trials suggest topiramate may be useful.

  C. **Opioid Dependence/Withdrawal:** Opioid withdrawal is characterized by nausea, emesis, stomach cramps, diarrhea, sweating, rhinorrhea, anxiety, muscle cramps, bone pain, and severe craving. Detoxification with methadone can alleviate the withdrawal syndrome. Clonidine is also helpful in reduction of withdrawal, but is not as effective as methadone. Adjunctive prochlorperazine (5-10 mg PO/IM q 6-8hr prn) is given for nausea/emesis; dicyclomine (20 mg PO q6hr) is given for stomach cramps or diarrhea; ibuprofen (600 mg po q6hr prn) is given for muscle or bone pain; and methocarbamol (500-750 mg q6hr prn) can help during the initial days of detoxification.

  D. **Nicotine Dependence:** Sustained-release bupropion has been approved for smoking cessation. Up to 50% of patients taking bupropion will achieve abstinence from tobacco after 12 weeks of treatment. This rate is twice the rate of placebo. Success of bupropion is increased by combining bupropion with a smoking cessation program. Varenicline (Chantix) is more effective than bupropion for smoking cessation based on one head-to-head study.

  E. **Sedative/Hypnotic Withdrawal:** Marked withdrawal symptoms can occur with abrupt discontinuation of sedative/hypnotic medications.

  F. **Psychostimulant Abstinence Syndrome:** Discontinuation of psychostimulants such as amphetamines, methylphenidate, and cocaine can produce fatigue, depression, hypersomnia, and irritability. Treatment usually consists of supportive care. Benzodiazepines can be used to treat irritability.

Acamprosate (Campral)

Category: Acamprosate is a synthetic compound with a chemical structure similar to homotaurine.
Mechanism: The exact mechanism of action is unknown. It may interact with glutamate and GABA neurotransmission.
Indications: Maintenance of alcohol abstinence.
Preparations: 333 mg tablets.
Dosage: 666 mg po tid, 333 mg po tid if renal impairment present.
Half-Life: 20-33 hours.
Clinical Guidelines: Efficacy in patients who currently abuse other substances has not been demonstrated. It should not be used until alcohol detoxification and alcohol abstinence has been achieved.
Adverse Drug Reactions: The most common side effects are diarrhea, nausea, headache, GI upset, rash, insomnia, asthenia, depression and anxiety.
Drug Interactions: Acamprosate does not inhibit cytochrome enzymes.

Buprenorphine (Subutex, Suboxone)

Category: Synthetic opioid.
Mechanism: Buprenorphine is a partial agonist at the mu-opioid receptor and an antagonist at the kappa-opioid receptor.
Indications: Treatment of opioid dependence.
I. **Preparations:**
    A. **Suboxone:** Sublingual tabs with buprenorphine 2 mg/naloxone 0.5 mg or buprenorphine 8 mg/naloxone 2 mg.
    B. **Subutex:** 2 or 8 mg sublingual tablets of buprenorphine.
II. **Dosage:**
    A. **Induction:** Induction should occur under physician supervision. Subutex should be used for induction when signs of withdrawal are present. To avoid precipitating withdrawal, patients may be given 8 mg of Subutex on day one and 16 mg of Subutex on day two. On day three and thereafter, Suboxone at a dosage of 16 mg per day is recommended.
    B. **Maintenance:** Suboxone is preferred for maintenance because it contains naloxone. The recommended target dose of Suboxone is 16 mg per day. Titration to the target dose should be accomplished by increasing the dosage by 2-4 mg per day to suppress opioid-withdrawal symptoms. The range is between 4-24 mg per day.
    C. **Half-Life:** 37 hours for buprenorphine; 1.1 hours for naloxone.
III. **Clinical Guidelines**
    A. In order to prescribe buprenorphine, clinicians need to be board-certified in addiction psychiatry or addiction medicine or have completed an approved 8-hour training course in the management of opioid-dependent patients.
    B. Subutex should be administered at least 4 hours after use of heroin or other short-acting opioids. It should ideally be administered when early opioid-withdrawal signs appear.

    C. There in minimal experience with transferring patients on methadone maintenance to buprenorphine, and withdrawal symptoms may occur during induction.

    D. Suboxone is preferred to Subutex for maintenance due to the inclusion of naloxone.

II. Adverse Drug Reactions

    A. Respiratory and CNS depression can occur with buprenorphine, especially if used intravenously. The risk of respiratory depression, including possible death, is increased if buprenorphine is combined with alcohol, benzodiazepines or other CNS depressants. Caution should be used in patients with compromised respiratory function, such as patients with chronic obstructive pulmonary disease.

    B. Buprenorphine produces opioid dependence. Withdrawal symptoms will occur if the drug is abruptly discontinued. The naloxone in Suboxone can cause marked opioid withdrawal if used intravenously or sublingually by opioid dependent patients.

    C. Buprenorphine may cause hepatocellular injury. Cases of hepatic failure, hepatic encephalopathy and other hepatic disease have been reported. Liver enzymes should be measured at baseline and periodically during treatment.

    D. Allergic reactions, characterized by rashes, hives and pruritis, may occur. Bronchospasm, angioneurotic edema and anaphylactic shock have been reported. Hypersensitivity to naloxone is a contraindication to Suboxone.

II. Drug Interactions

    A. CYP3A4 inhibitors, such as ketoconzaole, erythromycin and protease inhibitors increase the plasma levels of buprenorphine, and a decrease in the dosage of Subutex or Suboxone may be required.

    B. CYP3A4 inducers, such as carbamazepine and St. John's wort, may decrease plasma levels, and a higher dosage of buprenorphine will be required.

    C. There have been several reports of coma and death in patients taking both buprenorphine and benzodiazepines, often after self-injection of crushed buprenorphine. Therefore, buprenorphine should be used with caution in patients taking benzodiazepines or other sedative-hypnotics.

    D. Suboxone and Subutex tablets should be placed under the tongue until dissolved because swallowing reduces bioavailability.

Bupropion (Zyban)

I. Pharmacology

    A. Category: Unicyclic aminoketone antidepressant.

    B. Mechanism: Bupropion may alter dopaminergic and noradrenergic neurotransmission.

    C. Indications: Smoking cessation.

    D. Preparations: 150 mg sustained-release tablets.

    E. Dosage: 150 mg qod for several days, then increase dosage to 150 mg bid.

    F. Half-Life: 4-21 hr.

II. Clinical Guidelines: Bupropion is generally well tolerated. Efficacy compared to nicotine patches or gum is unknown.

III. Adverse Drug Reactions

A. **Most Common Side Effects:** Dry mouth, insomnia, dizziness, and arthralgias.

B. **Seizures:** Rate of seizures at doses up to 300 mg/day is 0.1%. Bupropion is contraindicated in patients with a history of seizures, head trauma, brain tumor or who are taking medications that significantly lower seizure threshold. Avoid use in patients with anorexia or bulimia because of possible electrolyte imbalances leading to seizures.

C. **Mania:** Bupropion can precipitate mania or rapid cycling and should be used with caution in patients with bipolar disorder.

D. Use caution in patients with hepatic, renal or cardiac disease.

E. **Neuropsychiatric:** In depressed patients, bupropion has been associated with psychosis and confusion. These symptoms abate with reduction or discontinuation of the medication.

F. **Pregnancy:** Category B.

IV. Drug Interactions

A. **Enzyme Inducers:** Enzyme-inducing agents, such as carbamazepine, phenobarbital, and phenytoin, may induce lower plasma bupropion levels.

B. Cimetidine may inhibit the metabolism of bupropion, leading to higher plasma levels.

C. Although bupropion is not metabolized via CYP2D6, it is a 2D6 inhibitor. Caution should be used when coadministering bupropion with other drugs metabolized by 2D6, such as quinidine or oxycodone.

Clonidine (Catapres, Catapres-TTS)

I. Pharmacology

A. **Category:** Antihypertensive agent.

B. **Mechanism:** Alpha-2-adrenergic receptor agonist.

C. **Indications:** Used for opioid withdrawal. It may also be used adjunctively for other withdrawal syndromes, such as alcohol or sedative/hypnotic withdrawal, to dampen noradrenergic symptoms.

D. **Preparations:** 0.1, 0.2, 0.3 mg tablets; clonidine TTS patch - 2.5 mg/ 3.5 cm^2 (0.1 mg/day), 5.0 mg/ 7.0 cm^2 (0.2 mg/day), 7.5 mg/ 10.5 cm^2 (0.3 mg/day).

E. **Dosage**

1. **Opioid withdrawal:** 0.1-0.2 mg po bid-qid with 0.1 mg q4hr prn (max 2.4 mg/day) or use a TTS patch along with po prn.

2. **Methadone withdrawal:** 0.1-0.2 mg PO bid-tid.

F. **Half-Life:** 12-16 hr.

II. Clinical Guidelines

A. Clonidine reduces the autonomic signs and symptoms of opioid withdrawal. It does not have an effect on craving.

B. Abrupt cessation of clonidine can lead to rebound hypertension, which can be fatal in rare instances. It should be tapered gradually over several days when discontinuing use.

C. Use caution in patients with a history of cardiac disease or Raynaud's Syndrome.

    D. Clonidine patches are designed to deliver the equivalent of 0.1 mg, 0.2 mg or 0.3 mg per day over one week. Patches should be changed weekly if necessary.

II. Adverse Drug Reactions: Hypotension, sedation, and dizziness may be severe. Fatigue, dry mouth, nausea, constipation, sexual dysfunction, insomnia, anxiety, depression, photophobia, rash and weight gain may occur.

III. Drug-Drug Interactions
    A. Potentiates the sedation associated with alcohol, barbiturates, and other sedative/hypnotics.
    B. Tricyclic antidepressants inhibit the hypotensive effects of clonidine.
    C. Antihypertensive agents increase the hypotensive effects of clonidine.

Disulfiram (Antabuse)

I. Pharmacology
    A. Category: Aldehyde dehydrogenase inhibitor.
    B. Mechanism: Leads to elevated levels of acetaldehyde with subsequent toxic effects.
    C. Indications: Alcohol dependence.
    D. Preparations: 250, 500 mg tablets.
    E. Dosage: 250-500 mg qhs.
    F. Half-Life: 60-120 hr.

II. Adverse Drug Reactions
    A. Sedation, fatigue, headaches, acne, impotence, rash, metallic aftertaste, and irritability are relatively common. These side effects usually disappear during the first few weeks of treatment.
    B. Hepatotoxic effects can occur, and disulfiram should not be used in patients with pre-existing liver disease.
    C. Peripheral neuropathy, optic neuritis, and psychosis are rare complications of treatment.
    D. If alcohol is consumed, patients will usually experience flushing, headache, nausea, vomiting, dyspnea, thirst, diaphoresis, hypotension, palpitations, chest pain, anxiety, blurred vision and confusion.
    E. In severe reactions, respiratory depression, arrhythmias, heart failure, seizures and death may occur. Treatment of a disulfiram-alcohol interaction consists of supportive therapy. The disulfiram-alcohol reaction may occur for up to 14 days after discontinuing disulfiram.

III. Clinical Guidelines
    A. The combination of disulfiram with an alcohol recovery program decreases the risk of relapse. Patients must be motivated to stop drinking, otherwise, they usually stop taking the drug or drink while taking it.
    B. Use caution in patients with a history of renal or hepatic disease, CNS disorder, hypothyroidism or over age 50. Baseline liver function tests and an ethanol level are recommended.
    C. Periodic monitoring of liver function tests is advised. Warn patients about dietary and over the counter preparations that may contain alcohol, such

as cough medication. Disulfiram is contraindicated in patients with severe cardiovascular or pulmonary disease.

III. Drug Interactions
  A. Isoniazid may cause ataxia and mental status changes.
  B. Metronidazole may precipitate psychosis.
  C. Disulfiram may increase levels of diazepam, paraldehyde, phenytoin, tricyclic antidepressants, anticoagulants, barbiturates, benzodiazepines, and anticoagulants.

Methadone (Dolophine, Methadose)

I. Pharmacology
  A. **Category:** Synthetic opioid.
  B. **Mechanism:** Opioid-receptor agonist.
  C. **Indications:** Detoxification and maintenance treatment of opioid addiction. Methadone can only be prescribed for treatment of opioid addiction in a federally approved treatment center. The drug may be continued if the patient is hospitalized for another reason.
  D. **Preparations:** 5, 10 mg tablets; 10 mg/mL solution.
  E. **Dosage**
    1. **Detoxification:** For short-term use (21 days maximum), the initial dosage is 10-20 mg po on the first day. Increase by 5-10 mg per day over the next few days, up to 40 mg per day in a single or divided dose. Maintain at this dosage for 2-5 days and then decrease by 5 mg qod.
    2. **Maintenance:** Treatment with methadone after 21 days is considered maintenance. A dosage of 40-80 mg is usually effective in preventing relapse.
  F. **Half-Life:** 24-36 hr.

II. Adverse Drug Reactions
  A. Methadone produces tolerance along with physiological and psychological dependence. Tolerance to the euphoric effects may lead to overdose. Overdose can lead to respiratory and cardiovascular depression, coma and death.
  B. The most common adverse reactions include sedation, nausea, emesis, dizziness, sweating, constipation, euphoria or dysphoria, dry mouth, urinary retention and depression.

II. Clinical Guidelines
  A. Use caution in patients with a history of respiratory disease, hepatic or renal abnormalities, seizure disorder or head injury.
  B. Women who conceive while on methadone should continue taking the drug; however, the newborn will require medical care for withdrawal symptoms.

III. Drug Interactions
  A. CNS depressants can potentiate the effects of alcohol, sedative/hypnotics, other narcotics, general anesthetics and tricyclic antidepressants.
  B. Desipramine may increase desipramine concentrations.
  C. Carbamazepine may lower plasma levels of methadone.
  D. **MAOIs:** The combination of an MAOI and meperidine and fentanyl have led to fatalities.

Naltrexone (Revia, Vivitrol)

I. **Pharmacology**
   A. **Category:** Opioid antagonist.
   B. **Mechanism:** Antagonist of opioid receptors.
   C. **Indications:** Alcohol dependence (reduces craving) and opioid dependence (blocks euphoric effects of alcohol).
   D. **Preparations:** 50 mg tablets; 380 mg injection.
   E. **Dosage**
      1. **Alcohol craving:** 50 mg/day or 380 mg every 4 weeks by IM gluteal injection.
      2. **Opioid abuse:** Start with 25 mg on first day; then 50 mg/day.
   F. **Half-Life:** 13 hrs (including active metabolite).

II. **Adverse Drug Reactions**
   A. Naltrexone may precipitate acute opiate withdrawal in patients who are still using opiates. Nausea is the most common adverse effect, which is minimized by starting with 25 mg qod or administering with food. Other adverse effects include insomnia, headache, anxiety, fatigue, dizziness, weight loss and joint and muscle pain.
   B. Naltrexone may cause hepatocellular injury when given in excessive dosages. It is contraindicated in patients with significant liver disease. Liver enzymes should be monitored. Oral naltrexone has caused hepatic injury with doses ≤ 5 times the recommended dosage. Oral injectable naltrexone carry and FDA black box warning regarding hepatoxicity.
   C. Injectable naltrexone may cause injection site reactions as well as side effects seen with oral naltrexone. May cause eosinophilic pneumonia, Depression and suicide occurred more frequently with injectable naltrexone than placebo.

II. **Clinical Guidelines**
   A. Naltrexone decreases the euphoria associated with alcohol consumption when used in combination with an alcohol treatment program. It reduces craving, and there are fewer relapses. Naltrexone also lowers consumption of alcohol if a patient relapses.
   B. The utility of naltrexone in opiate-dependent patients is more controversial. Some heroin dependent patients will attempt to use high dose of heroin in order to overcome the Mu receptor blockade. This can lead to accidental overdose and death by respiratory depression.
   C. Pregnancy category C.

III. **Drug Interactions**
   A. Patients who are currently using opioids will experience withdrawal due to the antagonist effect of naltrexone. If continued opioid use is suspected, a naloxone challenge may be given, and the patient is observed for signs of opiate withdrawal. Patients should be opioid free for at least 14 days before initiation of naltrexone.
   B. Naltrexone will block the analgesic effects of opioids, and greater than average doses of analgesics may be needed for pain relief.
   C. Disulfiram and naltrexone should not be combined because of the hepatotoxic potential of both of these agents.

Varenicline (Chantix)

I. **Mechanism:** Partial agonist of α4β2 nicotine acetylcholine receptors. Varenicline blocks the ability of nicotine to activate these receptors and stimulate dopamine, which is thought to be the mechanism that reinforces smoking and relieves nicotine craving and withdrawal.

II. **Indications:** Smoking cessation.

III. **Preparations:** 0.5 mg, 1 mg tablets.

IV. **Dosage:** Days 1-3: 0.5 mg qd. Days 4-7: 0.5 mg bid. Day 8 to the end of treatment (usually 24 weeks): 1 mg bid.

V. **Half-Life:** 17-24 hours.

VI. **Clinical Guidelines:** Patients should begin taking varenicline one week before smoking quit date. Patients who have quit smoking after 12 weeks should continue taking varenicline for 12 more weeks, then discontinue. Reduce the dosage in patients with sever renal impairment. Varenicline does not reduce the weight gain often seen with smoking cessation.

VII. **Adverse Drug Reactions:** Nausea, insomnia, abnormal dreams, abdominal pain, constipation, headache, vomiting, flatulence, dry mouth.

VIII. **Drug Interactions:** Cimetidine reduces renal clearance of varenicline and increased its serum levels by 29%. Increased side effects occur when varenicline is used in combination with nicotine patches.

References, see page 115.

Cognitive Enhancers

I. **Indications:** Reversible acetylcholinesterase inhibitors and NMDA receptor antagonists are used for the treatment of cognitive impairment associated with early Alzheimer's disease.

II. **Pharmacology**
   A. Cognitive impairment associated with Alzheimer's disease is thought to be caused by deficiency of cholinergic neurotransmission. Cholinesterase inhibitors result in increased synaptic concentrations of acetylcholine.
   B. While these drugs do not alter the overall course of the disease, they can prolong functional status in demented patients early in the course of the disease while there are still sufficient numbers of cholinergic neurons present.
   C. Memantine has a unique mechanism of action (NMDA receptor antagonist) and may work by decreasing glutamate medicated excitotoxicity.

III. **Clinical Guidelines**
   A. These medications improve cognitive performance in patients with mild-to-moderate dementia of the Alzheimer's type. Prior to treatment, patients should undergo a medical examination to rule out treatable causes of dementia.
   B. Cognitive function should be evaluated using standardized testing (eg, mini-mental status exam) prior to treatment and periodically thereafter to provide an objective measure of treatment response. Improvement of 1-2 points on the mini-mental status exam can be observed in patients with mild to moderate cognitive impairment. Mild-to-moderate disease is defined on the mini-mental status exam as a score between 10-26.
   C. Clinical studies indicate that improvement is temporary. Decline often is evident by 30 weeks. The rate of decline appears to be slower with acetylcholinesterase inhibitor treatment.
   D. Tacrine was the first acetylcholinesterase inhibitor, but it has essentially been replaced by newer medications, which do not carry the risk of hepatoxicity.

IV. **Adverse Drug Reactions**
   A. Due to increased cholinergic activity, gastric acid secretion can be increased, resulting in increased risk of ulcer development.
   B. Other predictable adverse effects caused by the cholinergic mechanism of action include nausea and vomiting, diarrhea, anorexia, weight loss, dizziness, syncope, and bradycardia. These tend to be dose related and can also be minimized slowly titrating the dose upward.
   C. Cholinomimetics may reduce seizure threshold, and exacerbate obstructive pulmonary disease.
   D. Tacrine is associated with liver toxicity.

Donepezil (Aricept)

I. **Indication:** Mild-to-moderate dementia of the Alzheimer's type.
II. **Pharmacology**
   A. **Class:** Piperidine.
   B. **Mechanism:** Reversible selective acetylcholinesterase inhibitor.
   C. **Metabolism:** Half-life is 70 hours; hepatic metabolism through CYP2D6 and 3A4 hepatic isoenzymes, followed by glucuronidation.
   D. **Preparations:** 5, 10 mg tablets.
III. **Clinical Guidelines**
   A. **Dosage and administration:** 5 mg qhs for 4-6 weeks, then increase to 10 mg qhs as needed. The 10 mg dose is associated with a higher incidence of side effect but may be more effective for some patients.
   B. **Pregnancy and Lactation:** Category C.
IV. **Adverse Drug Reactions:** May cause syncope and exacerbate bradycardia; most common are nausea, vomiting, diarrheas, insomnia, muscle cramps, fatigue and anorexia, which often resolved with continued treatment.
V. **Drug Interactions:** Minimal effect in regard to cytochrome P450 enzymes. Avoid or reduce dosage of beta-blockers to decreased incidence of bradycardia or syncope
VI. **Adverse Drug Reactions:** Most common are nausea, vomiting, diarrhea, insomnia, muscle cramps, which often resolve with continued treatment.

Galantamine (Reminyl)

I. **Indications:** Treatment of mild-to-moderate Alzheimer's dementia.
II. **Pharmacology**
   A. **Class:** Tertiary alkaloid.
   B. **Mechanism:** Reversible, competitive acetylcholinesterase inhibitor.
   C. **Half-Life:** 7 hours.
   D. **Preparations:** 4, 8 and 12 mg tablets; 4 mg/mL oral solution.
III. **Clinical Guidelines**
   A. **Dosage and Administration:** The recommended starting dose is 4 mg bid, increasing to 8 mg bid (16 mg/day) after 4 weeks of treatment. A further increase to 12 mg bid (24 mg/day) may be attempted after a minimum of 4 weeks at the previous dose. The recommended therapeutic dose for most patients is 16-24 mg/day.
   B. **Pregnancy and Lactation:** Category B.
IV. **Adverse Drug Reactions:** Bradycardia, nausea, vomiting, diarrhea, anorexia, weight loss, dizziness, syncope. Side effects tend to be cause by the cholinergic mechanism of action and are dose related.
V. **Drug Interactions**
   A. Galantamine is metabolized via CYP2D6 and CYP3A4; therefore, inhibitors of either of these cytochrome enzymes will reduce galantamine clearance. Paroxetine (2D6), erythromycin, nefazodone (3A4) and keto-conazole (2D6, 3A4) are inhibitors of these cytochrome enzymes.
   B. No clinically significant effects on digoxin levels or prothrombin time (in patients receiving warfarin) have been noted.

Rivastigmine (Exelon)

I. **Indications:** Mild-to-moderate dementia of the Alzheimer's type.
II. **Pharmacology**
   A. **Class:** Phenyl carbamate.
   B. **Mechanism:** Reversible selective acetylcholinesterase inhibitor.
   C. **Metabolism:** Rivastigmine is metabolized and eliminated by the kidneys. Because the dose is adjusted based on tolerability, adjustments in renally impaired patients are not always necessary.
   D. **Half-Life:** 1.5 hours.
   E. **Preparations:** 1.5, 3, 4.5, 6 mg capsules; 2 mg/mL oral solution.
III. **Clinical Guidelines**
   A. **Dosage**
      1. **Initial Dosage:** 1.5 mg bid, after 2 weeks increase to 3 mg bid.
      2. **Maintenance Dosage:** 3 mg bid may be effective. The dose can be increased if necessary to 4.5 mg bid, and then to 6 mg bid at two week intervals if required and if tolerated. May be given with food to reduce GI side effects.
   B. **Pregnancy Class:** Category B.
IV. **Adverse Drug Reactions**
   A. Most common side effects are nausea, vomiting, diarrhea, dizziness, anorexia, headache, abdominal pain and sedation.
   B. Rivastigmine has more peripheral effects than donepezil, which may result in more gastrointestinal side effects.
V. **Drug Interactions:** Minimal effect in regard to cytochrome P450 enzymes.

Tacrine (Cognex)

I. **Indications:** Mild-to-moderate dementia of the Alzheimer's type. Tacrine can be hepatotoxic and is rarely used.
II. **Pharmacology**
   A. **Class:** Acridine.
   B. **Mechanism:** Reversible non-specific cholinesterase inhibitor (inhibits both acetyl and butyl cholinesterase, increasing occurrence of systemic side effects).
   C. **Metabolism:**
      1. Extensive hepatic metabolism, principally by CYP 1A2 isoenzyme.
      2. Smoking reduces tacrine levels by induction of the 1A2 isoenzyme.
      3. Women develop blood levels 50% higher than men.
   D. **Preparations:** 10, 20, 30, 40 mg capsules.
III. **Clinical Guidelines**
   A. **Serum liver function** (ALT) should be monitored every two weeks for the first 4 months of treatment. If elevation is three times normal, the dose should be reduced. Elevations of more than five times normal, bilirubin above 3 mg/dL, hypersensitivity or jaundice require immediate discontinuation.

- **B. Dosage**
  1. **Initial Dosage:** 10 mg qid. After four weeks, the dose is increased to 20 mg qid. Daily dose is raised in 40-mg increments every four weeks to 120-160 mg/day.
  2. **Maintenance Dosage:** 120-160 mg/day in divided doses or qid.
  3. Tacrine should be administered at least one hour before meals because food impairs absorption.

IV. Adverse Drug Reactions
- **A.** Elevation of serum transaminases is the most frequent side effect (30%). This elevation appears to be reversible if tacrine is discontinued.
- **B.** Other side effects include nausea, vomiting, diarrhea, dizziness, agitation, anorexia, and confusion.

Memantine (Namenda)

I. Indications: Moderate-to-severe dementia of the Alzheimer's type.
II. Pharmacology
- **A. Class:** Dimethyladamantane.
- **B. Mechanism:** Memantine is an noncompetitive antagonist of the N-methyl-D-aspartate receptor. It reduces glutamate mediated excitotoxicity.
- **C. Metabolism**
  1. The majority of memantine is excreted unchanged in the urine.
  2. Memantine undergoes little if any metabolism via the cytochrome P450 enzyme system.
  3. There are no active metabolites.
  4. No dosage adjustment is required for patients over 65 years of age.
- **D. Half-Life:** 60-80 hours.

E. Preparations: 10, 20, 30, 40 mg tablets.
III. Clinical Guidelines
    A. Dosage: 5 mg PO q AM, then increase by 5 mg/week using bid dosing up to 10 mg PO bid.
    B. Memantine does not have the undesirable side effects associated with cholinesterase inhibitors.
    C. Cognitive improvement in patients with dementia treated with memantine is modest. Memantine may be used in conjunction with an acetyl-cholinesterase inhibitor to produce greater efficacy than either agent alone.
    D. Animal models suggest that memantine may have neuroprotective benefits.
IV. Adverse Drug Reactions
    A. Memantine is fairly well tolerated. Side effects include dizziness, headache and constipation in a small proportion of patients.
V. Drug Interactions
    A. Memantine does not significantly interact with CYP450 enzymes.
    B. Cimetidine, ranitidine, procainamide, quinidine and nicotine use the same renal cationic transport system and may increase blood levels of memantine.
    C. Co-administration of NMDA antagonists (amantadine, ketamine, dextro-methorphan) should be avoided. Such combinations could result in psychosis.
    D. Dopaminergic agonists and anticholinergic agents may be enhanced by memantine.

References, see page 115.

Antiparkinsonian Drugs

Psychiatric Side-Effect Management

I. **Indications:** Parkinsonian side effects are frequently encountered during treatment with typical antipsychotic agents and to a lesser degree with some of the atypical antipsychotics. Parkinsonian side effects includes tremor, rigidity, dystonias and akathisia.

II. **Pharmacology**

A. Parkinsonian side effects are thought to be mediated by blockade of nigrostriatal dopamine D2 receptors. They typically occur early after initiation of treatment with dopamine antagonists.

B. Antiparkinsonian drugs fall into two major categories:

1. **Anticholinergic drugs.**
   a. Benztropine (Cogentin).
   b. Trihexyphenidyl (Artane).
   c. Biperiden (Akineton).
   d. Procyclidine (Kemadrin).
2. **Dopamine agonists.**
   a. Amantadine (Symmetrel).

III. **Clinical Guidelines**

A. Anticholinergic agents are frequently required when treating patients with mid- and high-potency typical antipsychotics.

B. For patients being treated for the first time with mid- and high-potency antipsychotics, prophylactic treatment with an antiparkinsonian is recommended to prevent unpleasant extrapyramidal side effects. Prevention of these side effects can improve compliance with anti-psychotic medication.

IV. **Adverse Drug Reactions**

A. Anticholinergic agents can cause blurred vision, dry mouth, constipation, urinary retention, tachycardia and, less frequently, hyperthermia.

B. Elderly patients are more sensitive to anticholinergic agents and are at risk for developing anticholinergic induced delirium.

C. Anticholinergic agents are contraindicated in patients with glaucoma, prostatic hypertrophy, myasthenia gravis, or duodenal or pyloric obstruction. Benztropine is the least sedating anticholinergic agent.

D. Anticholinergic intoxication can occur if drugs with strong anticholinergic effects are combined. Confusion, agitation, hallucinations, ataxia, tachycardia, blurred vision, mydriasis, increased blood pressure, hyperpyrexia, hot and dry skin, nausea and vomiting, seizures, coma, and respiratory arrest can occur.

Amantadine (Symmetrel)

I. **Pharmacology**
   A. **Category:** Dopamine agonist.
   B. **Indications:** Neuroleptic-induced extrapyramidal symptoms.
   C. **Preparations:** 100 mg capsules; 50 mg/5 mL syrup.
   D. **Dosage**
   1. **Initial treatment:** 100 mg bid (max 400 mg/day). Perform trial off amantadine after 4 to 8 weeks to assess the need for continued use. Taper drug when discontinuing use.
   E. **Half-Life:** 24 hours, increased in elderly.
II. **Clinical Guidelines**
   A. Amantadine is useful when anticholinergics are contraindicated or ineffective. It is associated with less memory impairment than anticholinergics.
   B. Amantadine is less effective than anticholinergics in the treatment of acute dystonias.
   C. Dosage reduction is necessary in elderly or patients with reduced renal function.
   D. **Pregnancy:** Category C.
II. **Adverse Drug Reactions**
   A. Nausea (common), dry mouth, blurred vision, constipation, anorexia, hypotension, dizziness, anxiety, tremor, insomnia, irritability, impaired concentration, psychosis, seizure.
   B. Use caution in patients with a history of congestive heart failure and liver disease.
   C. Neuroleptic malignant syndrome has been reported with dose reduction or discontinuation of amantadine.
   D. Alcohol should not be used.
   E. Amantadine is contraindicated in patients with seizures.
III. **Drug Interactions**
   A. Anticholinergics may cause potentiation.
   B. CNS stimulants may cause irritability, seizure, and arrhythmias.
   C. Thiazides may increase the level of amantadine.
   D. Sympathomimetics may cause potentiation.

Benztropine (Cogentin)

I. **Pharmacology**
   A. **Category:** Anticholinergic (muscarinic receptor antagonist).
   B. **Indications:** Neuroleptic-induced extrapyramidal symptoms.
   C. **Preparations:** 0.5, 1, 2 mg tablets; 1 mg/mL soln. (IM).
   D. **Dosage**
   1. **Acute dystonia:** 1-2 mg IM (max 6 mg/day).
   2. **Chronic Extrapyramidal Symptoms:** 1-2 mg PO bid-tid. Perform trial off benztropine in 4 to 8 weeks to determine if continued use is necessary. Taper medication over 2 weeks.
   E. **Half-Life:** 3-6 hours.

II. **Clinical Guidelines:** Benztropine is the most widely used agent for extrapyramidal symptoms. Avoid using this medication with low-potency neuroleptics because of additive anticholinergic effects. Benztropine is contraindicated in glaucoma, prostatic hypertrophy, myasthenia gravis, duodenal or pyloric obstruction.

III. **Adverse Drug Reactions:** Drowsiness, dry mouth, blurred vision, nausea, weakness, confusion, constipation, urinary retention, sedation, drowsiness, depression, psychosis.

IV. **Drug Interactions:** Combining low-potency neuroleptics, tricyclics, and over-the-counter sleep preparations with benztropine may cause anticholinergic toxicity or anticholinergic delirium.

Biperiden (Akineton)

I. **Pharmacology**
   A. **Category:** Anticholinergic (muscarinic receptor antagonist).
   B. **Indications:** Neuroleptic-induced extrapyramidal symptoms.
   C. **Preparations:** 2 mg tablets.
   D. **Dosage**
      1. 2 mg PO bid-tid (max 6 mg/day). Perform trial discontinuation of biperiden after 4 to 8 weeks to determine if continued use is necessary. Taper medication over 2 weeks when discontinuing.
   E. **Half-life:** 4–6 hours.
II. **Clinical Guidelines:** Avoid using this medication with low-potency neuroleptics (additive anticholinergic effects). Biperiden is contraindicated in glaucoma, prostatic hypertrophy, myasthenia gravis and duodenal or pyloric obstruction.
III. **Adverse Drug Reactions:** Drowsiness, dry mouth, blurred vision, nausea, weakness, confusion, constipation, urinary retention, sedation, drowsiness, depression, psychosis. IV form is associated with orthostatic hypotension.
IV. **Drug Interactions:** Use of biperiden with low-potency neuroleptics, tricyclics, and over-the-counter sleep preparations may cause anticholinergic intoxication.

Diphenhydramine (Benadryl)

I. **Pharmacology**
   A. **Category:** Histamine receptor (H1) antagonist, muscarinic receptor antagonist.
   B. **Indications:** Neuroleptic-induced extrapyramidal symptoms, mild insomnia.
   C. **Preparations:** 25, 50 mg tablets; 25, 50 mg capsules; 10 mg/mL and 50 mg/mL soln. (IM, IV), 12.5 mg/5 mL elixir (PO).
   D. **Dosage**
      1. Extrapyramidal symptoms: 25-50 mg PO Bid, for acute extrapyramidal symptoms 25-50 mg IM or IV.
   E. **Half-Life:** 1-4 hrs.
II. **Clinical Guidelines:** Diphenhydramine is non-addicting and available over-the-counter.

III. **Adverse Drug Reactions:** Dry mouth, dizziness, drowsiness, tremor, thickening of bronchial secretions, hypotension, decreased motor coordination, GI distress.

IV. **Drug Interactions**
   A. The major concern about concomitant medication use with diphenhydramine is the additive effect of other sedatives and other medications with anticholinergic activity.
   B. MAOI use can prolong and intensify anticholinergic effects. Opiate addicts commonly add antihistamines to enhance the subjective effect of the illicit drug.

Trihexyphenidyl (Artane)

I. **Pharmacology**
   A. **Category:** Anticholinergic (muscarinic receptor antagonist).
   B. **Indications:** Neuroleptic-induced extrapyramidal symptoms.
   C. **Preparations:** 2, 5 mg tablets, 2 mg/5 mL oral solution.
   D. **Dosage:** Initially 1 mg qod, then increase to 2 mg bid-qid (max 15 mg/day). Perform trial off trihexyphenidyl in 4 to 8 weeks to determine if continued use is necessary. Taper medication over 2 weeks when discontinuing.
   E. Half-Life: 4-6 hours.
II. **Clinical Guidelines:** Avoid this medication with low-potency neuroleptics because of additive anticholinergic effects. Trihexyphenidyl is contraindicated in glaucoma, prostatic hypertrophy, myasthenia gravis and duodenal or pyloric obstruction.
III. **Adverse Drug Reactions:** Drowsiness, dry mouth, blurred vision, nausea, weakness, confusion, constipation, urinary retention, sedation, drowsiness, depression, psychosis. May cause restlessness and euphoric symptoms.
IV. **Drug Interactions:** Use of trihexyphenidyl with low-potency neuroleptics, tricyclics, over-the-counter sleep preparations) may cause anticholinergic toxicity or delirium.

References

References are available at www.ccspublishing.com/ccs

Selected DSM-IV Codes

ATTENTION-DEFICIT AND DISRUPTIVE BEHAVIOR DISORDERS

314.xx	Attention-Deficit/Hyperactivity Disorder
.01	Combined Type
.00	Predominantly Inattentive Type
.01	Predominantly Hyperactive-Impulsive Type

DEMENTIA

290.xx	Dementia of the Alzheimer's Type, With Early Onset *(also code 331.0 Alzheimer's disease on Axis III)*
.10	Uncomplicated
290.xx	Dementia of the Alzheimer's Type, With Late Onset *(also code 331.0 Alzheimer's disease on Axis III)*
.0	Uncomplicated
290.xx	Vascular Dementia
.40	Uncomplicated

MENTAL DISORDERS DUE TO A GENERAL MEDICAL CONDITION NOT ELSEWHERE CLASSIFIED

310.1	Personality Change Due to... *[Indicate the General Medical Condition]*

ALCOHOL-RELATED DISORDERS

303.90	Alcohol Dependence
305.00	Alcohol Abuse
291.8	Alcohol-Induced Mood Disorder
291.8	Alcohol-Induced Anxiety Disorder

AMPHETAMINE (OR AMPHETAMINE-LIKE)-RELATED DISORDERS

304.40	Amphetamine Dependence
305.70	Amphetamine Abuse

COCAINE-RELATED DISORDERS

304.20	Cocaine Dependence
305.60	Cocaine Abuse

OPIOID-RELATED DISORDERS

304.00	Opioid Dependence
305.50	Opioid Abuse

SEDATIVE-, HYPNOTIC-, OR ANXIOLYTIC-RELATED DISORDERS

304.10	Sedative, Hypnotic, or Anxiolytic Dependence
305.40	Sedative, Hypnotic, or Anxiolytic Abuse

POLYSUBSTANCE-RELATED DISORDER

304.80	Polysubstance Dependence

SCHIZOPHRENIA AND OTHER PSYCHOTIC DISORDERS

295.xx	Schizophrenia
.30	Paranoid Type
.10	Disorganized Type
.20	Catatonic Type
.90	Undifferentiated Type
.60	Residual Type
295.40	Schizophreniform Disorder
295.70	Schizoaffective Disorder
297.1	Delusional Disorder
298.8	Brief Psychotic Disorder
297.3	Shared Psychotic Disorder
293.xx	Psychotic Disorder Due to...
.81	With Delusions
.82	With Hallucinations
298.9	Psychotic Disorder NOS

DEPRESSIVE DISORDERS

296.xx	Major Depressive Disorder
.2x	Single Episode
.3x	Recurrent
300.4	Dysthymic Disorder

311	Depressive Disorder NOS

BIPOLAR DISORDERS

296.xx	Bipolar I Disorder,
.0x	Single Manic Episode
.40	Most Recent Episode Hypomanic
.4x	Most Recent Episode Manic
.6x	Most Recent Episode Mixed
.5x	Most Recent Episode Depressed
.7	Most Recent Episode Unspecified
296.89	Bipolar II Disorder
301.13	Cyclothymic Disorder
296.80	Bipolar Disorder NOS
293.83	Mood Disorder Due to... *[Indicate the General Medical Condition]*

ANXIETY DISORDERS

300.01	Panic Disorder Without Agoraphobia
300.21	Panic Disorder With Agoraphobia
300.22	Agoraphobia Without History of Panic Disorder
300.29	Specific Phobia
300.23	Social Phobia
300.3	Obsessive-Compulsive Disorder
309.81	Posttraumatic Stress Disorder
308.3	Acute Stress Disorder
300.02	Generalized Anxiety Disorder

EATING DISORDERS

307.1	Anorexia Nervosa
307.51	Bulimia Nervosa
307.50	Eating Disorder NOS

ADJUSTMENT DISORDERS

309.xx	Adjustment Disorder
.0	With Depressed Mood
.24	With Anxiety
.28	With Mixed Anxiety and Depressed Mood
.3	With Disturbance of Conduct
.4	With Mixed Disturbance of Emotions and Conduct
.9	Unspecified

PERSONALITY DISORDERS

301.0	Paranoid Personality Disorder
301.20	Schizoid Personality Disorder
301.22	Schizotypal Personality Disorder
301.7	Antisocial Personality Disorder
301.83	Borderline Personality Disorder
301.50	Histrionic Personality Disorder
301.81	Narcissistic Personality Disorder
301.82	Avoidant Personality Disorder
301.6	Dependent Personality Disorder
301.4	Obsessive-Compulsive Personality Disorder
301.9	Personality Disorder NOS

Index

Order Form

Current Clinical Strategies books can also be purchased at all medical bookstores

Title	Book	CD
Treatment Guidelines in Medicine, 2006 Edition	$19.95	$36.95
Psychiatry History Taking, Third Edition	$12.95	$28.95
Psychiatry, 2006 Edition	$12.95	$28.95
Pediatric Drug Reference, 2004 Edition	$9.95	$28.95
Anesthesiology, 2005 Edition	$16.95	$28.95
Medicine, 2007 Edition	$16.95	$28.95
Pediatric Treatment Guidelines, 2007 Edition	$19.95	$29.95
Physician's Drug Manual, 2005 Edition	$9.95	$28.95
Surgery, Sixth Edition	$12.95	$28.95
Gynecology and Obstetrics, 2006 Edition	$16.95	$30.95
Pediatrics, 2007 Edition	$12.95	$28.95
Family Medicine, 2006 Edition	$26.95	$46.95
History and Physical Examination in Medicine, Tenth Edition	$14.95	$28.95
Outpatient and Primary Care Medicine, 2005 Edition	$16.95	$28.95
Critical Care Medicine, 2007 Edition	$16.95	$32.95
Handbook of Psychiatric Drugs, 2008 Edition	$14.95	$28.95
Pediatric History and Physical Examination, Fourth Edition	$12.95	$28.95
Current Clinical Strategies CD-ROM Collection for Palm, Pocket PC, Windows, and Macintosh		$49.95

CD-ROMs are compatible with Palm, Pocket PC, Windows and Macintosh.

Quantity	Title	Amount

Order by Phone: 800-331-8227 or 949-348-8404
Fax: 800-965-9420 or 949-348-8405
Internet Orders: http://www.ccspublishing.com/ccs
Mail Orders:

Current Clinical Strategies Publishing
PO Box 1753
Blue Jay, California 92317

Credit Card Number: _____

Exp: ____ / ____

A shipping charge of $5.00 will be added to each order

Signature: _____

Check Enclosed _____

Phone Number: (_____)_____

Name and Address (please print):

_____

_____

_____

_____

1. Clozapine (Clozaril) is not associated with TD.
2. Aripiprazole (Abilify), olanzapine (Zyprexa), risperidone (Risperdal), quetiapine (Seroquel) and ziprasidone (Geodon) have a significantly reduced incidence of TD compared to the typical antipsychotics.

IV. Treatment
   A. Initial treatment should be continued for 4-6 weeks. If there is no response after this period, a change to an alternate medication is warranted.
   B. **Medically compromised patients**. Atypical agents are indicated in patients with conditions that predispose increased sensitivity to side effects of typical agents (eg, dementia).

V. Adverse Drug Reactions
   A. With the exception of clozapine the atypical agents are very well tolerated. There is a much lower occurrence of extrapyramidal symptoms.
   B. The atypical agents have a very low incidence of neuroleptic malignant syndrome and tardive dyskinesia.
   C. Type II diabetes and hyperlipidemia are associated with atypical antipsychotics (metabolic side effects).
   D. There is a suggestion from clinical trials in geriatric populations that risperidone and olanzapine are associated with an increased risk for ischemic stroke. Causality and generalization to other atypicals remains undetermined.
   E. The FDA has found that in the treatment of behavioral disorders in the elderly-demented patients, atypical agents are associated with increased mortality. The mechanism for this effect is unknown. They should be used with care in this population.

Aripiprazole (Abilify)

Class: Dihydrocarbostyril
Mechanism: Aripiprazole is a new partial agonist at the dopamine D_2 and the serotonin $5\text{-}HT_{1A}$ receptors, and it is an antagonist of the serotonin $5\text{-}HT_{2A}$ receptor.
I. Indications: Aripiprazole is indicated for the treatment of schizophrenia and acute mania. It should be considered for patients who have experienced metabolic side effects from other antipsychotic agents. It is also indicated for patients with tardive dyskinesia or severe side effects caused by other neuroleptics. Because of its relatively low liability for increasing weight, and serum glucose or lipids, it should be considered a first-line agent.
   Preparations: 2, 5, 10, 15, 20, and 30 mg tablets; 10 and 15 mg orally distinguishing tablet; oral solution: 1mg/mL; IM preparation: 7.5 mg/mL.
II. Dosage
   A. **Initial Dosage:** 10-15 mg qAM and increased to 20 to 30 mg per day after 2-4 weeks if needed.
   B. **Maintenance:** 10-30 mg per day.
   C. **Elderly:** While aripiprazole clearance is reduced by 20% in patients over 65, no dosage adjustment is required or recommended. Begin with a lower dosage in debilitated elderly patients.
III. Metabolism
   A. Half-life is 75 hours for aripiprazole and 94 hours for its active metabolite,

dehydro-aripiprazole. Hepatic metabolism is mainly through CYP2D6 and CYP3A4. Poor metabolizers who lack CYP2D6 have an 80% increase in aripiprazole plasma levels and a 30% decrease in dehydro-aripiprazole levels compared to normal.
  B. **Therapeutic Level:** Not established.
IV. Side-Effect Profile
  A. **Side effects** include headache, nausea and vomiting, which usually resolve within one week. The incidence of sedation is low but can occur at higher dosages. Anxiety and insomnia may occur, especially early in treatment. Akathesia can occur with higher doses and can sometimes be experienced as anxiety.
  B. **Orthostatic hypotension** occurs rarely. The incidence of extrapyramidal symptoms is comparable to placebo. Aripiprazole does not appear to effect QT_C intervals or serum prolactin.
V. Clinical Guidelines: Aripiprazole is usually given in the morning due to lack of sedation compared to other agents. Aripiprazole has a low liability for weight gain, or changes in glucose or lipid levels.
VI. Drug Interactions
  A. Coadminisration of aripiprazole with potent inhibitors of CYP2D6, such as quinidine, fluoxetine or paroxetine, can markedly increase blood levels (112% with quinidine) and requires dosage adjustment to one-half of its normal dosage.
  B. Ketoconazole or other potent inhibitors of CYP3A4 require adjusting aripiprazole to one-half of its normal dosage.
  C. Carbamazepine, a CYP 3A4 inducer, can lower plasma aripiprazole levels. The dose of aripiprazole should be doubled when co-administered with carbamazepine.
  D. Aripiprazole does not appear to effect levels of other cytochrome P450 substrates metabolized by CYP2D6,CYP2C9, CYP2C19, or CYP3A4.

Clozapine (Clozaril)

Class: Dibenzodiazepine
Mechanism: Multiple receptor antagonism occurs with the serotonin $5HT_{2A}$ receptor, and dopamine D1, D2, and D4 receptors.
Indications: Psychotic disorders that are refractory to treatment with typical antipsychotics. This agent is used for patients with tardive dyskinesia or severe side effects associated with other neuroleptics.
Preparations: 12.5 mg (unscored) 25, 100 mg scored tablets.
I. Dosage
    Initial Dosage: 25 mg bid, then increase by 25-50 mg every 2-3 days to achieve total daily dose of 300-600 mg. Dose may need to be given tid if side effects occur.
    Maintenance: 400-600 mg/day; some patients may require higher doses, but rarely more than 900 mg/day.
    Metabolism: Half-life 11 hours, hepatic metabolism, CYP1A2.
    Therapeutic Level: >350 ng/mL.
II. Clinical Guidelines
  A. Clozapine does not cause tardive dyskinesia or neuroleptic malignant